Praise for M

"Dr. Darria's witty, clever, and thoughtful approach to mothering advice will make you comfortable with the chaotic beauty of raising the most treasured friend you will ever have. Go get 'em!"

—Mehmet Oz, MD, Host, *The Dr. Oz Show*, attending physician, New York Presbyterian-Columbia University

"*Mom Hacks*, written from the heart of a mother and the scientific mind of a doctor, is a fun and informative read for busy parents. My favorite "hack" is Dr. Darria's wise advice about how moms can keep their own mind happy, even when their kids are draining. As a parent of eight and pediatrician for over fifty years, I highly recommend it."

—William Sears, MD, coauthor of *The Baby Book*

"*Mom Hacks* is a book every household should have to help maintain and improve the health of their children, and themselves. Dr. Darria fills the book with real medical lessons distilled from her years in the ER, as well as her own experiences as a mom of two children. This is the perspective and information moms everywhere need to hear, today."

—Sanjay Gupta, MD; CNN Chief Health Correspondent

"Dr. Darria—a mother, a doctor, and patient—is uniquely able to give 'insider' advice that's both relatable and trustworthy. Most importantly, her easily-absorbed hacks are a quick read on-the-go, can be read in any order, and are just what the doctor ordered for busy moms everywhere."

—Dawn Whaley, Sharecare President (and a mom)

"While we always hear 'it takes a village,' that's not always easy to find . . . until now. Welcome to your village of fun and sensible advice every mom needs to hear! Going from me to mommy wasn't the easiest transition for me, and I wish I had this book back then! It's a must-have for all of us navigating the wonderfully complicated journey of motherhood."

—**Lynn Smith, Mom and CNN Anchor**

"Dr. Darria delivers evidence-based bite sized tips to help the busy parent (including dads!) make the 'daily routine' simpler and gratifying."

—**Sudave Mendiratta, MD, FACEP; Associate Professor and Chair, Department of Emergency Medicine, University of Tennessee College of Medicine, Chief, Emergency Medicine, Erlanger Health System Chattanooga**

"Dr. Darria shares her wisdom and offers honest advice how moms can live their fullest, healthiest, and joy-filled lives while not sacrificing their most precious gift—their children. With balance, she reveals how we can have it all in *Mom Hacks*."

—**Meg Arnold, BSN, RN, and mom of four**

"*Mom Hacks* is a must-read for all moms to maximize beautiful moments with their children and minimize frustration. Combining the best in science with the honesty of a girlfriend, it's the all-in-one, laugh-out-loud book that is the exact information you'd get if your BFF were also a top physician and parenting expert."

—**Dr. Tanya Altmann, pediatrician, founder of Calabasas Pediatrics Wellness center, author of *Baby and Toddler Basics* and *What to Feed Your Baby*, and national spokesperson for the American Academy of Pediatricians**

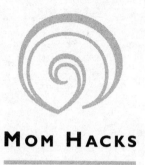

MOM HACKS

MOM HACKS

100+ Science-Backed Shortcuts to
Reclaim Your Body, Raise Awesome Kids,
and Be Unstoppable

Darria Long Gillespie, MD

Da Capo
LIFE
LONG

Da Capo Press
Hachette Book Group
1290 Avenue of the Americas, New York, NY 10104
www.dacapopress.com
@DaCapoPress

Printed in the United States of America
First Edition: February 2019

Published by Da Capo Press, an imprint of Perseus Books, LLC, a subsidiary of Hachette Book Group, Inc.

The Hachette Speakers Bureau provides a wide range of authors for speaking events. To find out more, go to www.hachettespeakersbureau.com or call (866) 376-6591.

The publisher is not responsible for websites (or their content) that are not owned by the publisher.

Print book interior design by Cynthia Young at Sagecraft.

Library of Congress Cataloging-in-Publication Data has been applied for.

ISBNs: 978-0-7382-8464-4 (hardcover); 978-0-7382-8463-7 (ebook)

LSC-C

10 9 8 7 6 5 4 3 2 1

To my beautiful babies:
You gave me the reasons I needed hacks
but also the fire to create them.
I love you more.

To BTG:
" . . . and it would not ring true.
If not for you."

To Mom and Dad:
Illegitimi non carborundum.

*Never allow a person to tell you "no"
who doesn't have the power to say "yes."*

—Eleanor Roosevelt

Contents

PART 1: NUTRITION 1

PART 2: EXERCISE 75

The Basics

Finding Time

Making It Fun

Finding the Motivation and Building the Habit

When the Going Gets Hard

PART 3: SLEEP 123

Sleep Foundation: Structure

Sleep Foundation: Routines

Sleep Foundation: Environment and Lifestyle

Relaxation and Cognitive Techniques for Sleep

Troubleshooting

Child-Specific Sleep Foundation and Troubleshooting

PART 4: RESILIENCE 187

My Days Are a Blur

Cracking Mommy Guilt and Self-Doubt

If You're Feeling Overcommitted and Exhausted

Nurture the Relationships that Nourish You

This book is designed to provide information and motivation about health and wellness. It offers helpful tips and education but is not intended to diagnose or treat any malady, or to replace, countermand, or conflict with the advice given to you by your own physician. If you have or think you have any health-care needs, you should contact a health-care professional and follow his or her advice. Information in this book is general in nature and is offered with no guarantees on the part of the author or Da Capo Press. Neither the author nor Da Capo Press is responsible for any specific health needs you bring, have, or might develop in the future, and we disclaim all liability in connection with the use of this book. Unless explicitly noted, the names and identifying details of people associated with events described in this book have been changed.

A Letter from Me to You

At seven months pregnant with my first child, I joked at dinner with an old friend (herself a mother of two), about "modifying" my running habit for my growing bump. I was caught off guard by her response: "Going to the gym. Yeah, that won't happen again after baby arrives."

I was stunned. And hurt. But was it true?

The Mom Epidemic

Shortly after that conversation, I was working on a news piece for mothers' health and learned that the truth wasn't pretty: For every child she has, a mother's risk of obesity rises by 7 percent. (I know. Where's the justice?) Moms are statistically more likely to have poor nutrition, get less exercise, have *waaaay* less sleep, and face alarmingly increasing rates of pregnancy-related complications and death in the United States.[1]

Suddenly, I was worried for moms. And for our children, whose generation may have shorter lives than our own. *What sort of Handmaid's Tale world was this?* Did we have to accept poor health as the cost of motherhood?

We find cures for cancer. We create artificial ears using 3-D printers. *We solved how to pee in space.* I knew we could figure this out.

I'd Found Solutions When I Was Told No Before—Could I Do It Again?

You see, I'd been here before, told my health as I knew it was going to change and that I had to live with it. When I was in medical school, I developed a large ovarian cyst. I awoke from emergency surgery having lost the entire ovary—and facing probable fertility problems. Within the next two years, I started to develop painful, swollen joints; I couldn't walk or see patients without pain. Within weeks, I went from daily runs to a low point when I realized my car was unlocked in downtown Boston—but was in too much pain to go back and lock it. I was eventually diagnosed with psoriatic arthritis and started weekly medication injections. They helped but came with their own risks (and if you need a laugh, watch a doctor learning to give herself an injection).

Statistics said that I probably wouldn't run or play piano at the same level again, certainly not without medications.

I did not like that answer.

So, I started to do research, and to make changes. A friend's father told me, "That'll never work."

It worked.

I was able to wean off my arthritis medications eight years ago. (Note: I'm not anti-medicine—I have huge faith in it. But, in my case—as for many—lifestyle plays a large role.) I gained control over the health outcomes I feared: I had two beautiful children. I resumed running. Most days, I can forget I have these diagnoses.

So, when my friend said, "You'll never . . . ," it was déjà vu all over again. And that meant it was time to get to work.

The Real Problem

Our bodies are amazing machines. They maintain an exquisite equilibrium: hormones, sleep, temperature, appetite, pH, and even millisecond-long variability between heartbeats are all under tighter control than the world's best stopwatch.

Except when they come undone. After observing my patients and mom friends, and becoming a mom myself, I realized the problem. Their equilibrium was off, and they were all caught in a vicious cycle of exhaustion, chronic stress, inadequate nutrition, cravings, weight gain, and low energy. Plus, they were overwhelmed by a barrage of conflicting health advice.

What Did Moms Need?

As an ER doctor, I must succeed amidst chaos. (*It sounds like a mom's typical day. It is*). To do that, we use a system of protocols, creative solutions, and training that let us be ready for anything.

So whatever comes through those ER doors, I can know "I've got this."

Suddenly, I realized that what moms needed was *not* more of the old advice that had long failed them; they didn't need suggestions to "use more willower" or "just try harder."

What Moms needed was a little more *I've got this*.

So, I took the skills and mindset that help me succeed in the ER and created a system to translate into daily life. I scoured the best science and incorporated environmental design, habits, and mindset change to make good health attainable—even unconscious. *Hacks don't add to your to-do list, they make it easier to do.*

So you can have a little more *I've got this*.

So you can be *unstoppable*.

How to Use This Book:
Choose Your Own Adventure

1. **Start with the section you want.** This book is broken into four sections: nutrition, exercise, sleep, and resilience. *For a kick-start, go to the Dr. Darria's Restore Diet (page 241).*

2. **Then choose *one* hack.** Start with just one hack and log it daily in the Hack Log (like the example at the end of this introduction). Feel free to experiment. You'll quickly see improvement and realize how good it feels to take back control with even the tiniest steps.

3. **Enlist your village.** For an even greater boost, enlist your family to join you—or at least cheer you on.

4. **Choose a theme song.** Because we all need a fight song. My current favorites are Shakira's "Try Everything" from *Zootopia* (apparently, I don't watch anything that's not Disney), Sia's "Never Give Up," and Sly and the Family Stone's "Role Model." Find my playlists at www.drdarria.com/momhacks (password: unstoppable), or find what makes your soul happy and play it with *abandon*.

What Does That Mean for Us All?

I'm grateful for my friend's comment that night because it catalyzed me to help moms—and myself. I probably wouldn't even change my arthritis, for that same reason. In which case, I guess you could call this book my *Lemonade*.

I walked off the airplane the other day with my infant's dirty diaper stuck to my sweater (pointed out to me by a kind bystander, God bless her). I don't claim to have everything figured out. But I have figured out things that work. Motherhood can feel like just barely treading water. But it does not have to cost us our health—or that of our children.

Perhaps you didn't dare dream that you could be an amazing mom, yet you are (or will be when baby arrives!). Perhaps you had no idea how beautiful and heart-expanding and *fun* motherhood could be. This book helps you have more of that. To have more energy, to achieve your body goals, to laugh, to just feel better. To be the mother and woman you want to be, on *your* terms. *It's time for a new mom world order.*

> *The question isn't who's going to let me; it's who's going to stop me.*
>
> **—Ayn Rand**

This is the book I wish I'd had that night at dinner. Now it's your book, for you to share with other mamas who need it. Don't listen to anyone who tells you motherhood has to be otherwise, and don't give up on yourself because I will not give up on you.

Godspeed, Mama,

Dr. Darria

Example Hack Log

(for a blank copy that you can print, and more great bonuses, go to
www.drdarria.com/momhacks [password: unstoppable])

WEEK 1	EXAMPLE RESPONSES
Hack Chosen	Walk 5 minutes every morning
How I plan to do it	I'll have my spouse watch children while I walk in the neighborhood for 5 minutes *Visualize the things you'll need to make this happen. Be realistic: if you see too many obstacles, make it shorter or simpler to start.*
Status of behavior on Day 0	I currently don't exercise at all
Day 1	✓ Did it!
Day 2	✓ Did it!
Day 3	✓ Did it!
Day 4	✓ Did it!
Day 5	✓ Did it!
Day 6	✓ Did it!
Day 7	✓ Did it!
Status of behavior on Day 7	I'm walking 5 minutes every day, and some days I even walk 10 minutes.
Have you noticed any other benefits?	I'm sleeping better, and I've noticed that I'm less tempted by a sweet snack at 10 A.M.

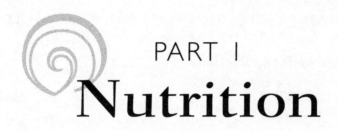

PART I
Nutrition

Make Healthy Eating Delicious

Design Your Life to Make Good Nutrition Easier

Getting the Whole Family Eating Well

Physicians at the beginning of the twentieth century were troubled by beriberi, a condition that afflicted their patients in Southeast Asia, triggering nerve problems, heart failure, and even death. In some regions, it killed as many as 50 percent of infants,[1] but doctors could not pinpoint the cause. Until Dr. Christian Eijkman suddenly noticed similar symptoms in his chickens after changing their feed to "polished" rice. For centuries, whole-grain rice had been a staple of the Southeast Asian diet, but, with the advent of rice processing machines, white rice supplanted it as the dominant food source.

The process of polishing the rice[2]—just as we see today with food processing—removed the vitamins. This deadly condition had arisen from a simple deficiency of thiamin (or vitamin B1). By restoring thiamin-rich foods and whole-grain rice to the diet, they "virtually wiped out the disease"[3] that had killed so many. *A deadly disease was solved with a simple diet change.*

Something similar happened in a research study of a cholesterol-lowering medication. Enough people were signing up, but Dr. Keith Roach, associate professor of clinical medicine at Weill Medical College of Cornell University, and his colleagues couldn't keep the participants in the study. The "problem"? After signing up, the research subjects were required to meet with a dietician. By following the dietician's guidance, 30 percent of the participants improved their health so much that they no longer needed the medication. By changing their nutrition, they had become too "healthy" for the study.[4]

Nutrition literally has the power to heal. Now, that can seem awfully high-minded when you're just trying to get your toddler to *eat*. The food that my daughter told me she loved yesterday "makes [her] tongue itch today." (What does that even *mean*? *That doesn't mean anything. It doesn't*.) They'd like more of whatever you ran out of yesterday, ThankYou VeryMuch. Plus, they sabotage your own diet by leaving you short on time, tired, and polishing off their leftovers at the kitchen counter. But there's hope.

A Word on Calories: Yes, Calories Still Count

Calories in − calories out = weight balance. That equation is basic physics: what goes in must come out *somewhere*, or it's stored as fat. But calories aren't *all* that matter—in fact, a slew of other factors, including what you eat, your hormone balance, and how your body responds, influence how many calories you take IN, and how readily your body burns them (OUT).

Which means that you can manipulate that equation for your benefit—or harm. (And that's no voodoo math.)

- **Food addiction and reward** (affects calories in). Certain foods stimulate the same reward center as addictive drugs, and food manufacturers spend millions designing new foods to do that even better. Not only do these foods trigger you to overeat; the more you eat, the more you crave, triggering a vicious cycle.

- **The impact of hormones** (affects calories in and out). You've likely heard of hormones such as leptin, ghrelin, insulin, and cortisol; when they're in balance, they keep the body running smoothly. But, when they're out of balance (like in many of us), they worsen the problem, triggering overeating and fat storage.

- **Food quality** (calories in, and a little out). Beyond just the calorie makeup, the quality of the food determines whether it gets plastered on our abdomen (hello spare tire) or gets used as energy.

P.S.: Apply some Zen to your toddler's eating. My second child is an adventurous eater, making mealtimes easy. My first is not, and I get the frustration that comes with that.

- Your job when it comes to your child's food:
  - to offer nutritious food,
  - to model enjoying it yourself.
- Your child's job: to eat it. Or not—her choice.
- Not included in your job description: letting her eat whatever she wants, being a short-order cook to accommodate her requests, or adopting hostage-negotiation tactics to coax her to eat.
- Although some children will immediately respond well to these hacks, others will take longer; and some little meal terrorists will resist entirely. It's not you, it's them. To the extent that you can, stay patient, keep consistent, breathe, and carry on.

For your own kick-start, start with the
Dr. Darria's Restore Diet (page 241).

The Science of Willpower
and Decision-Making

The latest research shows that willpower is a finite resource that easily runs out daily—so if you rely on willpower like most diets require, it's an automatic setup for failure.

The anatomy of willpower. Willpower comes from the brain region called the prefrontal cortex (PFC), which handles all of our executive functioning: abstract thinking, decision-making, and resisting temptation.

According to social psychologist Dr. Roy Baumeister, it's easy to overload the PFC and "drain" our willpower. Baumeister proved this in a study using freshly baked chocolate chip cookies . . . and radishes . . . because social psychologists are evil. Participants who had to sit in front of the cookies—but could only eat radishes—used all their willpower to follow the rules and gave up on the second challenge (a difficult math problem) in half the time—they simply ran out of willpower.

The PFC (sometimes referred to here as the "slow brain") can also be easily drowned out by the dominant fast brain, which is a primitive region focused on survival. Remember the *Saturday Night Live* "Sorority Girls" skit? Chris Farley is our fast brain, while David Spade is our slow brain/willpower. David Spade timidly asks, "Uh, I thought you were trying to lose weight?" and is crushed by a Chris Farley: "Lay off me, I'm **STARVING**!"

It doesn't have to be that way. In fact, we find that people thought to have high "self-control" don't actually have any more self-control than the rest of us; instead, they've just set up their life so that they face fewer temptations in the first place.[5]

Bottom line? *Don't bring David Spade as your backup to a Chris Farley fight, and don't try to rely on willpower alone when you're making health changes.* Instead, we'll make habit and environmental changes so that you're less exposed to temptation to begin with.[6]

Hacks to Set Your Goals

Hack 1
Find Your "Why"

If I told you right now to jump into oncoming traffic, you'd say no, right?

Now, what if I told you that you needed to do it to save your child? You'd be halfway into the street before I even finished the sentence.

The action was the same—but the difference? Meaning.

As an ER doctor, I've seen moms who have jumped in front of an attacking dog to protect their child, endured uncomfortable treatments in pregnancy for the sake of baby, and even one who carried her child to safety after a car accident before realizing that her other shoulder was dislocated.

We willingly take on any challenge—if the "why" is meaningful enough. The same goes for health decisions—people who successfully make major health changes have one thing in common: all are motivated by something meaningful to them, not just a jeans size or pounds on the scale. As Charles Duhigg puts it in *Smarter Faster Better*,[1] "If you can link something hard to a choice you care about, it makes the task easier."[2]

In other words, choose the true, meaningful outcomes of good nutrition to create that link between your food choices and your "why." Suddenly, you're no longer just deciding whether you want the donut enough to justify the calories, but whether you want it enough to jeopardize your energy to play with your children, your mental health, and even your children's future health. Linking it with your "why" makes it much more than "oh it's just a donut" and makes staying on track worth it—and easier. Choose two or three drivers from the list below that resonate with you.

- **A longer, vibrant life and more energy.** According to associate professor of clinical medicine at Weill Medical College of Cornell University Dr. Keith Roach, eating well can add five years to your life.[3] In research from Harvard, cleaning up just one meal a day reduced premature death by up to 17 percent.[4]

- **Lower risk of depression and anxiety.** People who eat a "Western" diet (high sugar/salt/saturated fat) are 60 percent more likely to develop depression.[5]

- **Better brain function.** Diets high in sugar and saturated fat increase inflammation, leading to oxidative damage in the brain. In children, a poor diet contributes to poor school performance, and possibly to attention and hyperactivity problems.[6] On the contrary, people who eat more produce have 20 percent greater productivity and 25 percent better job performance,[7] better memory, and a lower risk of dementia.

- **Fewer chronic medications.** Americans take more medications than people in any other nation,[8] which is caused in no small part by our diets. Changing your diet doesn't automatically mean you can stop medications, but sustained changes may significantly lower your need for them.

- **Lower risk of cancer.** Nutrition may cut the risk of cancer by as much as 30 percent.[9] An improved diet prevented prostate cancer recurrence as effectively as chemotherapy in one study[10] and may also be linked to lower breast cancer occurrence.[11]

- **Healthier gut.** A healthy diet also improves your microbiome, which impacts everything from weight to risk for asthma, allergies, and other autoimmune conditions. Plus, 95 percent of serotonin (a feel-good hormone) is produced in the gut, giving us even more reason to keep it healthy.

- **Healthy weight loss—and maintenance.** If you want to lose weight, then nutrition is the key. Of the more than 10,000 people surveyed who maintained significant weight loss, 98 percent had modified their food intake.[12]

- **To overpower your genes.** I have many patients who view their genes as a life sentence—not true! Your mother may have type 2 diabetes, your sisters may struggle to lose pregnancy weight, but hear this now: *Lifestyle trumps genetics.* Need proof? The weight of your best friend and your spouse (which reflect your lifestyle today) are more predictive of your weight than that of your parents.[13]

- **To make good health easier for your children—for life.** The foods we eat as infants and children impact our weight, preferences, and overall health years and even decades later. As one of the biggest influences on your child's early food preferences and habits[14] (no pressure, of course), the mind-set you model of nourishing your bodies will imprint on your children for life.

Hack 2
Choose Nutrition That
Work's with Your Body's Chemistry

Dietary fads seem to change every day, short on science and long on trendiness. Seeing my patients driven crazy (or worse, harmed) by what they read from a nutrition "expert" makes me want to dunk said expert in their own colon cleanse. It's just not right. (And by not right, I mean both the expert *and* the colon cleanse. Just *don't*.)

The problem with our current Western diet is that it's driven our body's equilibrium haywire. A good nutritional foundation will restore it and give you a way to eat for the rest of your life (as opposed to "dieting," which is unsustainable and miserable and should be fired). You'll have more energy, reach your body goals more easily, and even be able to sleep better.

You do *not* have to count grams or carbs or calories. You don't have to eat weird combinations or eliminate any one nutrient. In fact, a recent study showed that participants who simply prioritized whole foods—regardless of whether they ate low carb or low fat—lost weight and maintained it, without considering calories.[15] You'll also never have to eliminate any one macronutrient (such as carbs or fat) because as Dr. David Katz says, preventive medicine physician, founder of the Preventive Research Center at Yale University, and author of *The Truth About Food*, "If you focus on any given nutrient, . . . you're just inventing a new way to eat badly."

This will be the easiest nutrition guide you've ever read because it's simple: eat lots of "the best," moderate amounts of "the middle," and minimize or avoid "the ugly." But within that list, *you* get to choose what you love (and I'll give you many hacks to make it easier to work "the best" into your life and taste buds).

THE BEST: These are the building blocks of diets for the longest-living communities and should be the mainstay of yours, too.

Fruits and vegetables

Complex, whole grains

Beans

Legumes

Fish

Good fat (nuts, seeds, olive oil, avocados)

THE MIDDLE: Eat these if you want, in moderation (some long-living communities eat these, others don't).

Meat

Dairy

Wine

THE UGLY: Cut or minimize these.

Processed carbs/refined grains

Sugars

Trans fats (cut these entirely)

- **If you're looking for named diets for more details.** I like Mediterranean, Okinawan, and the DASH diet or Dr. Darria's Restore Diet (page 241). The vegan diet can also be healthy, but it can take more work to ensure you get enough of the required nutrients.

- **What don't I like?** There are many other "trendy" diets. Atkins or ketogenic diets may result in short-term (six- to twelve-month) weight loss but are tough to sustain *unless you actually like eating pork rinds 24/7.* Also, studies show that they may lead to elevations in cortisol and inflammatory markers,[16] and the high saturated fat content concerns me for its potential long-term vascular health impact. As for Paleo: it's better than the traditional American diet, but that's a low bar. The current branded Paleo diet lacks legumes and whole grains, and it is also a far cry from our ancestors' actual diet (which was low in saturated fat, took over 50 percent of calories from produce, and included up to 100 grams of fiber a day.[17] Which also means cavemen were very . . . um . . . *regular*. But I digress).

- How many servings? You'll notice that I don't usually give you a "limit to xx servings a week," because I don't expect anyone to keep track. Instead, focus more on how your plate is filled, following the "trifecta" rule (page 241), and you'll be just fine.

For a kick-start, start with the Dr. Darria Restore Diet (page 241).

The Building Blocks
of a Healthy Diet

Hack 3
Produce—How to Choose It

Fruits and veggies protect against everything from weight gain to cancer, chronic diseases to constipation (hey, that matters).

Every so often, I'll see people who are so hung up on buying organic that if they can't, they just won't get the produce. So let's just start by saying that *any* produce is better than none; because an out-of-season, conventionally grown cantaloupe is still without question better than fries, a steak, or . . . well . . . pretty much anything else you can buy. Got it? Good.

Now that we have that covered, use the list below when you want to get the biggest nutritional (and delicious) bang for your buck.

- **Eat produce in season.** In-season veggies tend to cost less and are fresher. (See table on page 15.)

- **Eat locally grown.** Locally grown produce is likely fresher and more nutrient rich than produce shipped from miles away. Plus, local farms tend to be smaller, so they typically need less pesticide. Try your farmer's market, local CSA (community-supported agriculture), or farm co-op for

13

fresh veggies in season. Not knowing what you'll get in a CSA box also encourages you to eat produce you may not otherwise try.

- **Seek brighter colors for more nutrients.** When comparing produce, the brighter the color, the more antioxidants, and the better it is for you. For instance, purple cabbage has more antioxidants than white. Also, produce often starts to fade as it ages, so the more vibrant colors may indicate freshness.

- **Frozen produce is a great alternative.** I always have frozen produce in my freezer; it's more convenient than fresh because it's prechopped, prewashed, and not going to go bad in five days. That means you can go from bag to pan with no prep. Also, because it's typically packaged right at peak freshness, frozen produce is often more nutrient rich than its fresh counterpart. Steam or microwave frozen veggies or toss them into a stir-fry or stew. I also keep frozen versions of my favorite smoothie staples (such as frozen kale, mango, or spinach) for when I'm out of fresh.

- **Throw in canned or jarred produce.** Canned produce such as corn, beets, and hearts of palm are great for sides or salad. Buy the low sugar/low sodium versions when possible, and rinse them well to reduce any excess sugar, salt, or starch. Jarred is also an excellent option for minced garlic (because I'm not mincing fresh garlic cloves when everyone's hangry), as well as beets, pickles, and raw probiotic-rich cabbage or sauerkraut.

FALL	**Veggies:** Beets, cauliflower, green beans, pumpkin, radishes, kale **Fruits:** Apples, figs, mangoes, pears, pomegranates, cranberries
WINTER	**Veggies:** Brussels sprouts, sweet potatoes, carrots, onions, winter squash, kale **Fruits:** Grapefruit, oranges, pineapple, pears, lemon, apples
SPRING	**Veggies:** Asparagus, avocado, broccoli, cabbage, rhubarb, spinach **Fruits:** Apricots, bananas, strawberries
SUMMER	**Veggies:** Avocado, beets, bell peppers, carrots, corn, cucumbers, eggplant, green beans, summer squash, zucchini, tomatoes **Fruits:** Watermelon, blueberries, blackberries, cantaloupe, honeydew, kiwi, mangos, peaches, plums, strawberries

Hack 4
Produce—How to Keep It Fresh and Ready to Eat

To be clear, a plastic bag in the produce drawer is where veggies go to die: An average family of four throws out about $1,600 worth of produce a year.[1]

When it's twenty minutes past dinnertime and your kids are starving, you're reaching for the fastest thing possible—and that usually isn't uncut/unwashed veggies. *Unless* you prep ahead. Then, new scenario: open fridge, grab chopped carrots and cabbage. Throw into pan with a can of baby corn, bag of frozen peas, and sesame oil. Stir-fry for five to seven minutes and done. Sha-zaam! Mom hero! (*Slow clap.*)

Liberate your veggies! *Vive le fruit!* Have produce ready for immediate consumption and you are more likely to actually eat it.

- **Weekend prep.** Take forty-five minutes to prep for the week, and you'll be thankful every day. Enlist children ages three and above (littles can help wash and dry or do things like break off asparagus ends). Your goal is to have *no* produce left in the grimy plastic storage bags. A few tips:

  - **Dry everything really well.** This is important, or it will get mushy. Then, place in the container with a dry paper towel to absorb excess moisture. If you see fluid collecting after a few days, drain it so the produce stays fresh.

  - **Store in clear glass containers.** Not only is it safer than plastic, it also allows you to easily see what's inside. Plus, it looks pretty, so you'll eat it.

> For more details, watch my veggie-prep hack video at
> www.drdarria.com/momhacks (password: unstoppable).

- **Totally okay cheat: Buy it prepped.** There's no shame in buying produce prechopped, especially when you're busy. It is more expensive, but it's better than throwing away produce you never had time to clean. I'll do this for tedious tasks, such as stir-fry veggies, so I can dump them into a pan in seconds.

Foods	Best Method to Prep and Store
Hearts of romaine lettuce, cabbage, celery, kale, asparagus	Wash carefully, trim ends, and store wrapped in paper towel inside storage container or plastic bag. You can also store asparagus by standing it in a small amount of water, like flowers.
Green/yellow/red peppers, carrots, melon, papaya, broccoli, cauliflower, green beans, radishes (leave radishes whole, but trim ends)	Chop into pieces and place in a glass container. (A spritz of lemon juice on fruit slows browning.) Dry peppers especially well before (and after!) you chop. Larger pieces tend to stay fresher and last longer than very small ones.
Berries, tomatoes, grapes, cherries	Rinse and place on top of a dry paper towel inside a glass container, or in a produce-specific container with an inner liner that elevates food off the bottom of the container.

Hack 5
Produce—How to Cook It

If your home-cooked veggies resemble your elementary school cafeteria lunch, it's no surprise that everyone in your family (including you, come on, we're being honest here) hides them under a napkin.

No more school cafeteria veggies. When you know the best ways to cook produce, you can win over the pickiest eaters. I know this because I live with one. When we first met, my husband informed me that he only ate fruits and vegetables that are orange: carrots, cantaloupe, and . . . (naturally) . . . oranges. And no, he was twenty-five, not five. That was more than a decade ago; last week he went back for seconds on my roasted mushrooms and green beans (Hallelujah, he's a changed man! *Does dance.*). If he can do this, so can you.

- **Pair with a little fat.** Not only does a little fat make produce taste um . . . *delicious,* it's necessary to absorb certain vitamins. So, add olive oil to your spaghetti sauce, hummus with crudité, olives or avocado to a salad, and salmon with leafy greens.

- **When in doubt, have a "veggie boost."** You can either count your servings of veggies per day (um, no), or you can have what I call a "veggie booster" such as a salad or smoothie every couple of days, so you know you're getting enough. If it's a snack or side, stick to only fruits, veggies, and ground flax or chia seeds to keep the calorie count reasonable. If it's the meal, add protein powder, Greek or almond yogurt, or nut butter to a smoothie, or protein, hummus, or nuts to a salad. Otherwise, experiment and throw in what you like!

Still Not Sure How to Cook?
Use This Handy Cheat Sheet

VEGGIES	COOKING	TIPS
Sweet potatoes (whole or sliced), eggplant, asparagus, beets, green beans, cauliflower, Brussels sprouts	**Roast/bake**	Toss with 1–2 tablespoons olive oil, sprinkle kosher salt, pepper, garlic, or rosemary. Heat oven to 425°F–450°F. Cook time varies by veggie and your oven (anywhere from 10 minutes [green beans] to 45 [potatoes]).
Beans, asparagus, cabbage, peppers, snap peas, zucchini, sliced carrots, baby corn, bok choy, edamame, water chestnuts	**Stir-fry**	Chop into relatively uniform pieces. **Sauce:** (1) sesame oil and either low-sugar teriyaki sauce or low-sodium soy sauce or (2) a low-sodium chicken stock, a little white wine (a little in the pan . . . a little in my glass) and a teensy bit of Worcestershire sauce. Heat pan to high, then add veggies in small batches, stirring constantly.
Broccoli, cauliflower, carrots, green beans, artichokes, spinach	**Steam**	Cut uniformly. Place 1 inch water in a large pot and boil (add lemon juice for flavor). Add veggies in a steamer insert. Sprinkle after cooking with olive oil, herbs, and spices.

(Continues)

(Continued)

Still Not Sure How to Cook?
Use This Handy Cheat Sheet

VEGGIES	COOKING	TIPS
Green beans, asparagus spears, carrot sticks, green peas, sugar snap peas	Blanch	Place veggies into a pot of rolling boiling water. Boil until al dente (2–4 minutes). Immediately place in ice bath to stop cooking process. Eat as a side, serve as a crudité platter, or add to your salad.
Carrots, spinach, cabbage, zucchini, mushrooms, kale	Sauté	Bring 1–2 tablespoons olive oil to medium heat. Add chopped veggies. Stir often (but not constantly, to allow for browning). For Brussels sprouts: Blanch to take out bitterness, then sauté in olive oil, garlic, herbs (tarragon, parsley), and very little salt.
Fresh or frozen green peas, green beans, broccoli	Microwave	Pour frozen veggies into a glass bowl, and heat about 2 minutes. Pour out any melted water, add olive oil, a little shredded parmesan, and herbs.

Hack 6
Make Your Family a "Longevity Salad"

When husband and I first started dating (Clearly the downside of being married to me is that I share your food habits with the world. I'm like the Taylor Swift of health.), he would force himself to eat a salad of iceberg lettuce, carrots, cheese, croutons, and fat-free Italian dressing. I finally had to break it to him—the sad salad that he dreaded wasn't even good for him.

So I asked him whether I could make him a salad one night. If he didn't like it, he could always go back to his own. Enter, [drumroll] . . . the Longevity Salad! *I called it that because we were just dating and I wanted to impress him; I didn't have any other culinary skills at that point besides making salad.* (Ask me someday about my fondue explosion or my "spaghetti meat tartare" . . .) But the name fits: not only is it good for you and full of superfoods, it's also rich in flavor and has a delicious good-for-you dressing (so, unlike the sad salad that makes you question life, eating the Longevity Salad actually makes you also WANT to live longer).

- **Rule #1: There are no rules.** Which makes that the only rule. Throw in anything from the list below; there are no required magical combinations or proportions. Experiment. Add what you like, leave out what you don't.

- **Use these items to make mini "salad bars," so family members can make their own salads.** Set everything out in the containers you prepped over the weekend, and let everyone customize their own salad, which young children particularly enjoy.

Longevity Salad 1-2-3-4

START WITH A BASE:	Spinach, romaine, iceberg lettuce, arugula, or endive
Add Your Veggies	Peppers (I love yellow, red, and orange)
	Tomatoes (mini grape tomatoes, large heirloom, or anything in between)
	Sugar snap peas or green peas
	Avocado (refrigerate the remainder along with the seed and a spritz of lemon juice to delay browning)
	Sprouts
	Beans (chickpeas, red beans)
	Corn (canned is fine)
	Carrots
	Beets (canned or jarred is fine)
Optional: Add fruit	Small chopped apples, pears, or grapes
	Dried fruit (high in sugar, so use in small amounts)
Optional: Add crunch	A (small) serving of nuts
	Water chestnuts
	Mung bean sprouts
	Jicama
Optional:	Add a protein, if this is your full meal

Top Your Longevity Salad with a Delicious Homemade Vinaigrette

½ cup really good balsamic vinegar (my favorites are from the specialty food stores and are really thick)

2 teaspoons finely minced garlic (I outsource mincing by buying the jars of minced garlic, in the refrigerator aisle)

1 tablespoon Dijon mustard (I also like Dijonnaise)

¼ cup water

1½ tablespoons olive oil

Optional: 1–2 teaspoons lemon juice to taste

Optional: 1 teaspoon of dried basil, oregano, or parsley

Hack 7
Carbs—Choose the Best Carbs

You get a carb! *You* get a carb! *Everybody gets a carb!* It's Oprah's next giveaway, I swear. Or at least it should be because a license to eat carbs is as great as getting a free car.

In the past two decades, carbs have gotten a bad rap, causing many of us to fear them while we simultaneously crave them, *which makes things . . . well, awkward.* Here's the issue: there are *good* carbs, and there are *not-so-good* carbs. Black beans are carbs, as are broccoli, quinoa, and papaya. But so are pancakes, white pasta, and jelly beans.

Good carbs are necessary; in fact, they're linked to lower rates of obesity and cancer, plus longer life spans. So, you can eat carbs. Just aim for *good* carbs.

- **Opt for low-glycemic-load carbs.** You've probably heard of the glycemic index, but a new and better measure of carbs is actually glycemic load (GL). A lower GL better stabilizes our blood sugar, helps us feel full, and reduces insulin resistance and weight. In fact, a Harvard study showed that a low-GL diet keeps your metabolism revving better than a low-fat diet.[2] You don't need to memorize it—just stick to the best and good carbs in the table.

- **When you do consume carbs, eat them with protein or fat.** Even the best carbs still cause blood sugar to rise, so eat them with a little protein or fat to slow absorption. Have oatmeal with a handful of walnuts or top whole grain toast with avocado and scrambled eggs/egg whites, or nut butter.

The Best	The Middle	The Ugly
Beans and Legumes: Kidney, black beans, garbanzo, pinto, lentils	Whole wheat/grain pasta	Table sugar
	Oatmeal (not instant)	White bread
Nonstarchy Fruits and Vegetables (most fall into this category)		Juices
	Ancient grains: Barley, bulgur, spelt	Sugar-sweetened beverages
Cereals Made with 100% Bran		
	Brown rice	White rice
Ancient Grains: Couscous, Quinoa		White pasta
	Starchy vegetables: Corn, sweet potatoes	French fries
Sprouted/Whole Grain Bread		Sugary cereals
		Candy

Hack 8
Fat—Add Good Fats Back to Your Diet

I remember sitting in the lunchroom in high school with my cross-country teammates, thinking we were so healthy while we ate plain baked potatoes, bagels with fat-free cream cheese, and bowls of fat-free frozen yogurt. Was it any wonder that my body broke down and developed a stress fracture in each leg?

Fat makes for a popular fad: it was public enemy #1 for two decades, and now it's done a complete 180, with some "experts" hailing it as a miracle nutrient (*kind of like denim on denim being back in fashion, which worries me for our country*). The reality? Somewhere in between.

Is low fat to blame for the obesity crisis?

Everyone went low-fat crazy in the 1990s, but obesity continued to climb. Those two facts have led to many singling out a reduced-fat diet as the culprit. It was not. The problem was not that we went low fat. Had we gone low fat by eating naturally low-fat whole foods such as produce and lean meats, we would have been fine. We didn't do that. We instead ate processed Frankenfoods that were low-fat chemistry experiments. (The food industry loved the "low-fat craze.") And we ate a lot of it, drastically increasing our intake of added sugar and calories— and our waistlines.

Bottom line

It's not the absence or presence of fat that makes a diet healthy; it's the types of foods, including the types of fats. There are good fats and not-so-good ones, so use the table below to know what to choose.

Where Does Saturated Fat (Including Butter, Ghee, and Coconut Oil) Fall?

So, your BFF drinks ghee in her coffee every morning and adds butter and coconut oil to everything—but is that actually *healthy?* What's the skinny on saturated fat?

Studies have undeniably shown that people who consume more saturated fat have higher levels of bad cholesterol, inflammation and heart disease, and shorter life spans. So you don't want unlimited amounts of saturated fat.

Is there a difference between the saturated fat from animals (like beef) and from vegetables (like coconuts)? There likely is, but we don't know that for certain, and we don't know by how much. So, in the meantime, opt for what fats we KNOW are healthier, and have saturated fat only in limited amounts. And tell your best friend to replace the ghee with salmon, almond butter, or an omega-3 supplement for a healthier fat.

THE BEST: Monounsaturated Fats—make these the dominant sources of fat in your diet	
	Olives and olive oil
	Avocados and avocado oil
	Tree nuts (almonds, cashews, pistachios, pecans, hazelnuts, macadamia nuts)

THE GOOD: Polyunsaturated Fats—these should be the secondary sources of fat	
Polyunsaturated Fats—Omega 3s	Cold-water fish (salmon, mackerel, lake trout, herring, albacore tuna, sardines, anchovies) Walnuts Flaxseeds Tofu Grass-fed beef and "wild game" (antelope, wild venison, bison)
Polyunsaturated Fats—Omega 6s	**Note:** Although polyunsaturated fats are necessary, we tend to already eat too many of them in processed foods and restaurant dishes. So you don't need to seek *more* of these. Vegetable oils (corn, soybean, sesame [which is about half mono- and half polyunsaturated], sunflower) Walnut oil Tub margarine (some may be a combination of poly- and monounsaturated fats)
THE NOT-SO-GOOD: Saturated Fats—limit these in general	
Saturated Fats	Butter Dairy (milk, cheese, full-fat yogurt) Coconut and coconut oil Palm oil Beef, chicken skin

(Continues)

(*Continued*)

> **THE UGLY:** Trans Fats—eliminate these. Period. For every 2 percent of your calories from trans fats, you're raising your risk of heart disease by 23 percent.

Trans Fats	Commercially baked goods (cookies, cakes)
	Deep-fried foods
	Margarine (stick form)
	Anything with the words "partially hydrogenated oil"
	Note: Some trans fats occur naturally in meat and dairy. Those aren't as bad as the manufactured trans fats in this list.

- **Cook with high-smoke-point oils.** The higher the smoke point of a fat, the less it is oxidized (i.e., releases free radicals into your food) by high heat. Fats with high smoke points include extra virgin olive oil (particularly if cold pressed), avocado oil, high-oleic sunflower oil, macadamia nut oil, and coconut oil.

Hack 9
Heal Your Microbiome

You have 100 trillion little *Lactobacillus*, *Bacteroides*, and *Bifidobacterium*[3] in your gut right now (I know. They're so cute, right?), and *their* health is linked with *your* risk of asthma or autoimmune conditions,[4] as well as the state of your emotions, weight, and stress response.[5] Researchers found that the microbiome of obese mice differed from that of lean mice, and, when they transplanted an obese mouse's microbiome into a lean mouse (just go with me and avoid the gross visual), the lean mouse became obese,[6] and the obese mouse became thin. Studies have even found that an unhealthy microbiome in infancy increases a child's risk of being overweight seven years later.[7]

Unfortunately, antibiotics, industrialized life, and processed foods mean that our microbiomes are drastically different from those of our ancestors.[8]

- **Eat your probiotics.** Probiotic foods contain good bacteria and can help repopulate a healthy microbiome[9] in adults and children.[10] There isn't a set recommended amount, so just incorporate a few servings a week. Good sources include unsweetened yogurt (look for labels designating multiple bacteria strains, made from whole milk, organic or grass fed, and possibly vat pasteurized[11]), kefir, fermented vegetables such as sauerkraut and kimchi, natto (a popular Japanese dish), organic salted gherkin pickles, and brine-cured olives.

- **Eat foods high in prebiotics, to feed your microbiome.** Prebiotics are the fuel for good bacteria. Prebiotic-rich foods are high in insoluble fiber and include fruits, berries, seeds, raw onions, raw garlic, and Jerusalem artichokes.

- **Consider supplements in some cases.** For general health, the best way to get probiotics is still via our food. However, probiotic supplements may be helpful for specific conditions such as irritable bowel syndrome,[12] peptic ulcer disease, and possibly eczema[13] and colic in children. They also can be effective in preventing antibiotic-associated diarrhea,[14] so when my children or I need antibiotics, I also give a probiotic. Always check with your pediatrician or doctor first and give the probiotics at least two to three hours apart from the antibiotic, to avoid any interaction.

Other Ways to Nurture Your Microbiome

- **Use antibiotics cautiously.** Widespread use of antibiotics, from prescriptions to antibiotics in our food, harm our good bacteria and nourish the bad gut bacteria. Be a good antibiotic steward: take antibiotics only when truly necessary (no, not at the first sign of a cough or runny nose), finish the *entire* course, and opt for antibiotic-free meats and dairy.

- **Don't be afraid of germs.** The Hygiene Hypothesis suggests that we may have more allergies and autoimmune conditions because we've overly disinfected our lives. Use hand sanitizers sparingly and only when you don't have access to soap and water. When home, avoid antibacterial soaps except around food and raw meats. Plus, because studies show that children who grow up with a dog in the house or on a farm have significantly lower rates of asthma,[15] make sure your kiddos have plenty of outdoor time (and say yes to the pooch, if you want one).

Hack 10
Eat the Right Protein

Protein is the trendy diet's friend, and for good reason: it increases fullness and keeps blood sugar level. But, just like fat, the source of the protein determines whether it's healthy or not. For instance, people who eat large amounts of red meat are at greater risk for heart disease, cancer, and mortality,[16] while replacing animal protein with plant-based protein lengthens life span.[17]

Does that mean you should avoid red meat entirely? Not necessarily. A study from *JAMA* showed that if you maintain a healthy lifestyle, the occasional red meat (two servings a week or less) is okay.[18]

THE BEST: Make these sources the mainstay of your diet

Beans and legumes. A study in the *Journal of Obesity* showed that a daily serving increased satiety.[19] So, start a weekly meatless night tradition: in a study where people didn't know whether they were eating a bean-based burger or a meat-based one, the bean-based version was reported as more filling and just as delicious.[20] Cook veggie, quinoa, mushroom, or soy-based proteins the same way you'd cook your meat-based versions, and don't tell anyone it's meat-free until *after* they've licked their plates.

Nuts and seeds. Eating peanuts, tree nuts, and walnuts five or more times a week is linked to a lower risk of heart attack and stroke.[21]

Fish. Fish consumption is associated with lower rates of heart disease. If you're nursing or pregnant, limit consumption to two servings a week, and only those species that are lower in mercury. (See the Environmental Working Group's Seafood Calculator[22] for the database I kept close at hand when I was pregnant.)

Poultry. White meat is the best, as it's lower in saturated fat. If you prefer dark meat, remove the skin. Although "hormone-free" labels on chicken are a gimmick (it's illegal to give hormones to chickens we eat), it may be wise to select "antibiotic-free" or "pasture raised."

Soy- or grain-based products such as quinoa. Like beans and legumes, these are a good source of protein and fiber.

(Continues)

32

(*Continued*)

THE MIDDLE: Have these if you wish, but in moderation

Dairy. Dairy products are rich in protein, calcium, and vitamin D. If you enjoy it, dairy can have a place in a healthy diet, although it's not necessary (many cultures, such as the long-living Okinawans, eschew dairy).

Eggs. Yes, you can eat eggs. (Seriously! Would I yolk about this?) The latest guidelines from the American Heart Association no longer restrict cholesterol in our food because it has only a minor impact on blood cholesterol levels for most people. However, eggs do have saturated fats (in addition to good fats), so intake still needs to be within limits.

Lean meats. When you're wanting red meat or pork, choose leaner cuts, which will have lower levels of saturated fat. Look for grass-fed beef or game (such as antelope or bison), which will have higher levels of omega-3s (good fat), and opt for hormone- and antibiotic-free options.

THE BAD AND THE UGLY: Avoid these

Processed meats. Steer clear of processed meats, including bacon, processed ham, hot dogs, and sausage.
If you do want to have these, opt for those that are nitrate- or nitrite-free but still eat only in small amounts.

What Not to Eat

Hack 11
Avoid Beverages That Sabotage
Your Metabolism

Mom always told me that "water is the drink of the wise man and woman." It turns out she's paraphrasing Henry David Thoreau (which I just found out. How did I not know this for 30 years?), and they're both correct. Our bodies are 60 percent water, and it's necessary for everything from maintaining our blood volume to electrolyte balance and organ function. Plus, research shows that people who successfully maintain weight loss most commonly drink water.[1]

The problem with sweetened drinks is that they're nothing but an empty calorie add-on because our brain doesn't register calories from beverages the same way it does calories from food. Eating a 250-calorie sandwich will decrease your appetite, but drinking those same 250 calories in a beverage won't. That's why sweetened beverages do a number on your weight and also your metabolism, hormones, and taste preferences.

- **Bottom line, drink more water.** Most of us shortchange our water intake and, because we confuse thirst for hunger, end up eating when we're actually thirsty. That explains why

33

people who drink more water consume fewer calories.[2] As a general rule, the number of ounces you need per day equals your weight divided by two. So, a 140-pound woman should aim for 70 ounces of water a day (age, activity, overall health, and heat/humidity also affect individual needs).

- **Make water more appealing.** Add slices of your favorite fruits or veggies to enhance your water (anything works, from oranges to cucumbers to strawberries). For a little extra bubbly, go for sparkling water.

- **Cut out sugary drinks.** A Johns Hopkins study showed that simply cutting out one sugar-sweetened beverage a day caused participants to lose weight.[3] You can do that. Start by replacing one sugary drink a day with tap or sparkling water.

- **Be cautious with artificial sweeteners.** "Diet" drinks and artificial sweeteners are a mixed bag. Although I still consider them better than sugar-sweetened drinks, they're not a free pass. In fact, they may be linked to weight gain by disrupting your microbiome and triggering your sweet tooth. Bottom line? A little here or there is fine—particularly if you're using them as a bridge to break a sugary-drink habit—but try to limit their regular use. If you use sweetener in your coffee, one study found it easier to just cut sweetener cold turkey than to slowly decrease the amount.[4] (Besides, if you take your coffee black, people assume you're a badass.)

- **Make water your child's primary beverage.** Children do not need juice, particularly when 12 ounces of "all natural, not from concentrate, no sugar added" apple juice has the same amount of sugar[5] as a can of soda (10 teaspoons).[6] Also, according to the American Academy of Pediatrics, unless your children are participating in "prolonged, vigorous sports participation or other intense physical activity," they don't need sports drinks, either.[7] Reserve juice and sports drinks as a treat, and, even then, dilute it ⅓ juice to ⅔ water.

Hack 12
Minimize Endocrine Disruptors in Food Storage

Would you like a side of plastic with your meal?

If you're eating something that came wrapped in fast-food-type plastic wrappers or that was heated in plastic, you're also having a helping of chemicals along with it. And that can significantly impact your health. Chemicals like BPA, phthalates, and other plastics are considered "endocrine disruptors" that impact hormone regulation and metabolism and contribute to obesity, diabetes, and other chronic diseases. BPA exposure increases fat growth in infancy and can even affect weight decades later.[8]

The biggest source of our exposure to these chemicals is food containers, including plastic bottles and sippy cups, can linings, takeout packages/wrappers, plastic storage containers, and receipts. These chemicals seep into our food directly or rub onto our hands and transfer to food when we touch it.

- **BPA-free or BPA-alternative is *not* good enough.** When we discovered the dangers of BPA, the market responded with a host of "BPA-free" plastic products. Except, now we're learning that BPA-free alternatives are just as harmful.[9] The best way to avoid them is to minimize your use of plastic containers and plates, period.

- **Instead, use glass or stainless steel whenever you can.** As much as possible, I store and serve food and beverages in glass or stainless steel (a plastic lid is okay). That includes sippy cups and bottles—glass or metal versions are more expensive, but they're more durable and won't melt in the dishwasher. I've also bought little caps that you can attach to your glass baby bottles, converting them to sippy cups. Yes, the caps are made of plastic, but it's much less plastic than an entire sippy cup.

- **Avoid plastic in the dishwasher.** Unless a plastic piece has touched meat or dairy (or is just gross), I try to wash plastic by hand. Minimize putting plastics in your dishwasher, as the high heat makes chemicals seep out of the plastic and onto your other dishware.[10] Plastic can also melt into the dishwasher, causing damage—plus an awful burning smell.

- **Microwave in glass or china.** Never heat foods in plastic containers, particularly thin takeout containers. Transfer to a glass or microwave-safe china plate.

- **Avoid cutesy plastic plates.** A cute Minnie Mouse plate may be tempting, but these cutesy plastic dishes are another source of these chemicals. As soon as your child is old enough to not throw dishes on the floor, swap them to adult china.

- **Limit receipts and wash hands after handling them.** Receipts are laden with BPA, and we often grab the receipt when we get takeout, food from the grocery store, or fast food and then use that same hand to handle our food. Decline the receipt if you don't need it or wash your hands before touching food. Definitely also keep receipts away from children, particularly infants and toddlers who love to nom nom on anything they touch.

Note: For more details on brands and types of containers that I suggest, see my recommendations and what I use at www.drdarria.com/momhacks (password: unstoppable).

Hack 13
Break the Processed Food and Sugar Habit
Step 1: Cutting Hidden Sources

The Science of Sugar

To our caveman ancestors, sugar represented a quick source of energy, so they evolved to crave it. That was okay because sugar was rare at the time and naturally coexisted with other nutrients, such as fiber, vitamins, minerals, protein, or complex carbs. So, even when our ancestors craved sugar, it was hard to come by and came in small concentrations.

But in the past two hundred years, that all changed. We can now mass-produce foods that are nothing but straight sugar. Suddenly, we could get a hit of the sweet stuff in its most concentrated form—whenever we wanted it.

THE DIRECT EFFECT OF SUGAR

Our bodies aren't made to work that way. Here's what's supposed to happen: you eat a small amount of sugar, your blood glucose rises, and your body releases insulin, which helps your body utilize the glucose. Blood glucose levels then decrease, insulin levels return to normal, and everyone's happy.

However, if you're constantly eating sugar (which most of us are, thanks to sweets and even hidden sugar foods), your blood glucose is always elevated, and your insulin stays high, signaling your body to store glucose as fat (so not cool insulin, not cool). That's why diets high in sugar lead to obesity, diabetes, cancer, and even premature aging.

(Continues)

(Continued)

THE INDIRECT EFFECT OF SUGAR:
THE SUGAR DEPENDENCE CYCLE

But wait! There's more (isn't there always?). Sugar also triggers our brain's "reward zone," the same area where drugs and alcohol act.[11] Every time you eat sugar, you make your reward zone happy—and it expects more. The more you eat, the more you crave it again—fast. Food manufacturers know this and spend millions yearly studying brain scans to identify the "bliss point": that perfect ratio of sugar, salt, and fat that are truly irresistible and completely override our normal fullness mechanisms. We crave more—and even feel withdrawal when we don't get it. It's like a designer drug—in an easy-open package.

Stress makes it even worse. If your stress levels are chronically high, your cravings worsen and your body simultaneously switches into fat storage mode. You're constantly hungry, overwhelmed by cravings, and storing more fat. No matter how much you give into your cravings, you never feel better.

Is that you?

If so, then it's time to break the sugar-dependence cycle.

Adults today get up to 25 percent of their daily calories from added sugar, which is oh . . . *five* times higher than the WHO's recommendation. According to researchers at the University of California, San Francisco (UCSF), 74 percent of grocery store foods contain added sugar:[12] obvious sources, such as candy, soda, and cookies, but also unexpected sources, such as processed foods, salad dressings, pasta sauce, BBQ sauce.

Remember how I said that part of the problem is constant sugar intake? Hidden sugars in your marinade and salad dressings (and everywhere else) keep your taste buds awash in sugar.

They train your brain to constantly expect and crave sugar, even when you're eating regular, non-dessert foods. (Plus, they're a bolus of extra empty calories.)

Researchers at UCSF, studied the effects of added sugar by limiting added sugar for children participating in a study. They let them eat "normal kid foods"—in fact, they ate pizza, hot dogs, and even bagels—just without added sugar. In nine days, their blood pressure and cholesterol improved, and they lost weight—even though the kids were encouraged to eat the same amount of calories. *Nine days!*[13]

So, step 1 of breaking your sugar-induced disequilibrium is to cut foods with hidden sugars. Dr. David Katz calls this "taste-bud rehab" and told me, "Taste buds are adaptable little fellas; when they can't be with the foods they love, they learn to love the foods they're with. . . . It absolutely doesn't take very long . . . to reshape your palate."

Note: Decoding sugar on nutrition labels. The FDA has proposed changes, but they won't go into effect until 2020 at the earliest.[14] So, you'll need to become a label supersleuth.

- **Scrutinize labels of the most common culprits.** Common hidden sugar sources include salad dressings, pasta sauce, barbeque sauce, yogurt, cereals, child-specific foods (child-targeted cereals have 85 percent more sugar than those for adults[15]), frozen meals, and granola bars.

- **Label check #1: Look for sugar in the top five ingredients.** Sugar goes by many names, so look for all of these: dextrose, glucose, fructose, high fructose corn syrup (essentially anything ending in "-ose"), honey, molasses, agave, or corn syrup. If any of these is in the top five ingredients, save that food for dessert.

- **Label check #2: Look at grams of added sugar.** Although not all labels show this,[16] but for those that do, keep in mind that daily limits of sugar for men are 36 grams, 25 grams for women and children (that's per *day*).[17]

- **Buy unsweetened versions.** When you buy nut butters, regular or nondairy milk, oatmeal, applesauce, and other foods, choose unsweetened versions.

- **Make your own.** Many of the hidden-sugar culprits can be made in healthier versions easily at home: I make my own salad dressing (see hack #6), and pasta sauce can be made with tomatoes (canned or fresh), olive oil, garlic, onions, and various herbs. Also, replace sugary yogurts with plain yogurt and add just a small amount of honey or jam yourself—you'll add far less than the manufacturer would.

- **Naturally occurring sugar is okay.** Unless you suffer from diabetes or prediabetes, naturally occurring sugars in whole fruits are okay—our obesity epidemic did not arise from people eating too many strawberries.

Hack 14
Break the Processed Food and Sugar Habit Step 2: Cutting Obvious Sources

Once you've reduced the hidden sources of sugar, you may notice your cravings weakening, which means you've started to kick the habit. Now, it's time to go after the obvious sources. (I like to cut hidden sugars first because that makes the transition easier as your cravings decrease naturally.) Even if you come from a family of sweet tooths, a recent study showed that our environment and habits can impact our taste preferences just as strongly as genetics.[18] You can break the habit.

I'm not saying that you can *never* have sugary foods. (Please, don't we know each other well enough by now?) But, I want to help you break your *dependency* on them so you're eating them because you *choose* to do so, and not because you *need* them.

- **Replace processed carbs with whole ones.** Replace your highly processed carbs (including bread, rice, pasta, and even crackers), with complex ones: whole grain, quinoa, chickpea-based, or other protein-rich grains. Ease the transition with pasta and rice by mixing in ¾ of your regular version and ¼ of the whole grain and slowly increasing the whole-grain ratio.

- **Quit melt-in-your-mouth chips.** Food manufacturers design chips to have a soft, melty texture that your brain doesn't register for fullness. (Scientists call this "vanishing caloric density." Food manufacturers call it "*ka-CHING!*") A 2011 study in the *New England Journal of Medicine* found that the biggest weight-gain culprits were potato chips and French fries.[19] Make life easier for yourself, and keep these out of the house while you're breaking this cycle.

- **Say "no" to sugary snacks.** While you're breaking the habit, keep any sugary treats to a minimum, if not cold turkey. Head off afternoon cravings with an apple and one teaspoon of unsweetened nut butter or cheese, or hummus and unlimited carrots. Be sure to hydrate with plain water, too.

- **Find the reason.** We often crave a sugary food when we're not even hungry but are instead wanting a break or are stressed or bored. Try to address that need, instead of just covering it up with food. Is it a mental break? A reward after a good (or hard) day? Write up a list of rewarding nonfood activities: playing music (which triggers the same brain reward centers as food), taking a walk or a five-minute work break, calling a friend, or doing a fun activity with the kiddos. You'll likely distract yourself from the craving, plus research shows that even if you do eat the craved food in the end, if you've boosted your mood by taking these steps first, you'll still eat significantly less.[20]

- **Control portion size and enjoy.** If you want to have something sweet, remember that it's a treat, and that it is okay to have—in moderation. Portion yourself a single serving onto a plate, put away the remainder (ideally, somewhere out of reach), then, for goodness sakes, go *enjoy* it.

Hack 15
Watch Out for a "Lite" or "Fat-Free" Label Backfire

The label "lite" or "diet" is the kiss of death: these labels alone affect how delicious and filling (or not) we think a food is.

In one study, participants were given two samples of the same milk shakes with one labeled "nonfat/low calorie" and the other "rich." The *only* difference between the two samples was the label. After drinking the lite-labeled sample, the unwitting participants reported it as less filling than the rich-labeled version. But the unbelievable finding was that their levels of the hunger hormone Ghrelin were also higher after the lite-labeled sample—meaning that the *label even influenced their body on a biochemical level* (i.e., it wasn't "all in their head").[21]

- **Minimize low-fat/nonfat versions.** Foods that are manufactured to be low fat or fat-free have consistently higher amounts of sugar and carbohydrates than their original versions.[22] In fact, research shows that eating low-fat foods is associated with eating more sugar, carbs, and calories overall.[23] You're not even home-free with sugar-free diet versions, as the artificial sweeteners not only disrupt your microbiome but also enhance your sweet tooth and exacerbate future cravings.

- **If you want a food, choose a small portion of the regular, over the lite.** Researchers at Ghent University gave participants the same cheese several times, but when the same cheese was labeled "light," participants rated it as tasting inferior to the sample labeled "regular."[24] Stick to the real/original version instead of its manufactured, fat-removed counterpart, and you'll be satisfied with less.

- **Beware the "health halo" effect.** In a study in the journal *Appetite,* when female students were told that the cookies offered were healthy, they ate 35 percent more.[25] When we think something is lite or healthy, we subconsciously compensate by either eating more of that food or more of something else.

For a kick-start, start with the Dr. Darria Restore Diet (page 241).

Make Healthy Eating Delicious

Hack 16
Embrace New Flavors

I remember being at brunch in medical school when a friend said, "I'm not sure what flavor I want for breakfast today—sweet or savory?" Excuse me? I thought the decision was pancakes or waffles; I'd never thought in terms of flavor and its impact.

It turns out that there are five categories of flavors: sugar and salt (Western diet staples), and sour, bitter, and umami (my personal favorite). Not only do the latter three flavors boost taste, they also make us feel full more quickly.

Ayurvedic medicine, one of the world's oldest health practices, originating from India, suggests incorporating as many flavors as possible into any meal for balance, health, and a rich, multidimensional taste.

- **Combine flavors for a richer experience.** Combining multiple flavors drives us to eat more (which explains why you can't put down salty/sweet/sriracha kettle chips). Combine flavors to make healthier, whole foods more enticing.

  - Add umami flavors such as seaweed, pickled vegetables, tomato paste, or cured meats to vegetables, whole grains, or meat and fish for a warm, hearty taste.

- Tone down bitter foods, such as eggplant, by roasting them with a little olive oil and very little salt to enhance natural sweetness.
- Add citrus to brighten otherwise milder foods, such as a splash of lemon juice on fish, or a little lime on guacamole or papaya.
- Serve a salad with a tangy dressing.
- Play with flavor combinations for roast veggies by adding a salty/rosemary flavor one night, sautéing with olive oil and garlic the next, or seasoning them with a tangy Asian flavor another night.

The Three "Forgotten" Flavors

SOUR. Sour foods include lemons, fermented foods (yogurt), vinegar, wine, and some fruits like strawberries.

BITTER. Bitter foods include many of the leafy green vegetables (spinach, kale, radicchio); spices (such as turmeric, oregano, or rosemary); eggplant and zucchini; green, black, or most herbal teas; and coffee. Bitter foods can be great add-ons to mellow out a sweet or rich meal.

UMAMI. Umami refers to a savory/smoky/hearty flavor. Find it in mushrooms, seaweed, miso soup, cured meats, tofu, cheeses (especially like a hard-aged parmesan), tomatoes, or fermented foods such as soy sauce.

- **Follow flavor to help a craving.** Want something sweet? Go for a papaya, juicy mango, or honeydew melon. Tend to crave salty? I keep low-sodium cans of soup or "just add water" cups of dry miso soup at work, or hearts of palms at home. Or flip the script entirely by eating something with a clashing flavor: foods that cleanse the palate, such as grapefruit or a strong mint can short-circuit the craving (brushing your teeth also works this way).

Hack 17
Eat for Satiety

Satiety is our body's way of telling us when we've had enough. But it's easily manipulated by two factors: the satiety threshold, namely how much of any one food you need to eat to feel full, and sensory-specific satiety, which says that the more flavors and textures you're offered, the more you'll eat.

Sugar has a very high satiety threshold, which means that you have to eat a lot of it to feel full. The food manufacturers who want to make a sale know this. It's time you did, too, because these are crucial factors for how satisfied you feel after eating.

- **Eat foods high on the satiety threshold.** Unlike sugar, the flavors of umami, sour, and bitter all have a lower satiety threshold. So do lean proteins, foods with high water content (think fruits and some veggies), and those with lots of air (such as popcorn). Eat those foods to fill up without overeating.

- **Watch sensory-specific satiety with unhealthier foods.** Ever been entirely full at the end of dinner, then suddenly have space for dessert? Blame sensory-specific satiety: When you feel like you can't eat another bite of the main course, your brain actually reads that as fullness from those *specific foods*. So, when you're offered an entirely different flavor and texture—such as dessert—you suddenly have "room." The more food texture and flavor we're offered, the more we eat—up to 60 percent more.[1] So, when you have many options (say at a buffet or party), you're better off having decently sized portions of *fewer* foods (or just one dessert), rather than "just trying a little of everything."

- **Find healthy foods that are powerfully flavored.** Play with flavor further by adding these strong tastes to enhance the satiety of whole foods:

Mustard	Olives
Hummus	Fresh herbs and spices
Aged balsamic vinegar	Tomato paste
Low-sodium soy sauce	Chicken stock
Salsa (the spicier the more satiated you'll feel)	Capers
	Olive tapenade
Guacamole	Pesto
Sun-dried tomatoes	White bean puree
Garlic	Marinated tofu
Hard parmesan cheese	

Hack 18
Eat Mindfully

How often has this happened: You're watching TV after dinner and grab a bag of chips. The next thing you know, the bag is empty, but you don't feel full. In fact, you don't even remember the satisfaction of eating the chips.

It's called mindless eating, and we're all guilty of it. When you're distracted, you don't taste flavors as intensely[2] and don't register feeling full. So you overeat while also feeling less satisfied: a lose-lose situation.

Enter mindful and intuitive eating, which teaches us to listen to our body, to eat only when we're hungry, and to pay attention to how we feel while we're eating. Studies show that it leads to feeling more satisfied despite eating less, and it may improve our health and weight.

- **Before you eat, pause.** Take thirty seconds to be thankful for the people who worked to bring the food to you (the farmer, the truck driver, the waiter, the produce stocker at the store). Say a blessing or grace if you wish. Do this with your family as well—not only will it help everyone eat more mindfully, it creates a moment to slow down and pause amidst our busy day.

- **Practice *hara hachi bu*.** It takes ten to twenty minutes for your body to register your stomach's fullness, by which point you've easily overeaten. *Hara hachi bu* is a traditional Japanese principle that teaches you to stop eating when you're 80 percent full. Do periodic "gut checks" at your next meal to listen to your body.

- **If you're eating a treat/dessert, be sure to savor it.** What's worse than eating something indulgent, but so mindlessly that you didn't even enjoy it? That's madness! When you do have dessert or a treat, for the love of holiness, please savor it. Not only does it make you happier, it can satisfy you with less.

- **Minimize distractions when you eat.** Bright lights, loud and fast music, and the TV all lead us to overeat. Turn off the TV for meals. If you're going to eat a snack while watching TV, pour out the portion you want to eat and put away the rest because you know you'll be distracted.

Design Your Life to Make Good Nutrition Easier

Hack 19
Make Unhealthy Eating Inconvenient

Our great-great-great-grandmothers didn't need much will-power because they didn't have donuts . . . or 64-ounce soda slushies. And if Jane Cavewoman wanted to eat at 10 P.M. to bury her emotions about her Neanderthal (literally) boyfriend, she'd have to face nighttime predators just to find a snack. Our cravings are no different today, but our environment is.

We evolved to survive in an environment where finding calories was hard and physical activity was inevitable. But in the past 150 years, our environment changed: now, food—especially high-calorie, high-dependence food—is everywhere, while exercise is rare. Our brains and bodies are just not equipped for it. It's like we're cavewomen living in a modern-day world.

The same thing happens today when people from a country with a traditional diet and low obesity immigrate to the United States—in no time they've developed obesity, diabetes, and the risk of a shorter life span.[1]

But remember what I told you in the introduction: people who make the healthiest decisions do so not because they have a superpower but because "they do not put themselves in the position where they have to resist temptation as often."[2] They simply make their environment less tempting, and you can, too.

- **Don't keep it in the house.** In surveys of people who maintained long-term weight loss, 80 percent report not keeping tempting foods in their home. If eliminating all junk food incites a rebellion at home, keep some, but simply reduce the number of options (especially for those foods that you cannot stop eating).

- **Rearrange your pantry and fridge to move the unhealthy out of sight.** The grocery store knows you'll grab what's at eye level—and the same happens in your pantry. If the first thing you see is chocolate, every pantry trip becomes an exhausting exercise in willpower. For those indulgent foods that do stay, keep them on the highest shelf, out of sight and out of reach. Researchers at Utrecht University found that when chocolate was moved just out of reach, study participants ate 70 percent less—without extra cravings.[3] Put junk food high enough that you don't see it and need a stool to reach it, and you'll eat less without even trying.

- **Restrict where eating occurs.** When you eat in many locations (at the kitchen counter, in front of the TV, in the car), your brain links each of those locations with food, meaning they each trigger cravings. Reduce those brain linkages by limiting where your family eats to, say, the kitchen table.

- **Put the unhealthy options in opaque containers.** This would never work, right? Wrong. In a study from Ohio State, people ate 58 percent less M&Ms out of opaque containers than they did from clear ones.[4] Monkey see, monkey eat. Monkey no see . . . monkey no eat!

- **Don't store snacks with serving utensils.** Dr. Traci Mann does this in her own home with Rice Krispies treats, as she relays in *Secrets from the Eating Lab*. If you have a cake on the counter, keeping the knife with it only increases the chance that you'll slice off just a teensy sliver . . . ten times a day. Instead, cut yourself a reasonable portion, put the knife in the dishwasher, and enjoy the amount you served yourself.

- **Redirect your route to avoid a tempting stop.** If there's a specific cupcake shop (or a snack pantry at work) that is particularly tempting to you, stop trying to face these temptations head-on. Instead, find a route that avoids the area altogether.

Hack 20
Make Healthy Eating Convenient

The more tired and stressed we are (which is, well, every day), the more our willpower is exhausted and the more likely we are to take the easiest option. Research shows that if the healthy options are the easy ones, our brain—with its desire for convenience, will more frequently select them—without requiring any willpower.

Think it sounds too easy? Google employees were eating a *lot* of candy; to help everyone with their health, researchers suggested making a change: still have everything available, but put healthy snacks in clear jars, and place the M&Ms and other candies in opaque containers. That's all they did. The M&Ms were still as accessible, they just weren't on display in all their colorful chocolatiness. It worked. Over seven weeks, the 2,000 employees ate 3 million fewer calories from M&Ms.[5]

Yes. We humans really are that predictable.

- **Put the healthy in sight.** Once you've moved the junk food out of sight, swap healthy options into your pantry and fridge. What you see is what you (and your family) eat. In one study where researchers told families to put produce at eye level in the fridge but *did not ask them to change what they ate,* families automatically ate significantly more produce.

- **Put healthier options in clear containers.** Now that you put the junk food in opaque containers, take all the veggies and fruit that you prepped and put it in clear glass containers. The sight of them in your refrigerator is a reward for your weekend produce prep, serves as a visual inventory, and makes them more enticing.

- **Have produce available and within reach at all times.** Have hand fruit (apples, pears, plums) washed, dried, and placed on the counter in a bowl, so they're within reach of all members of the family. Your independent toddler who wants to get a snack all by herself can take anything from the fruit bowl.

- **Stock your fridge with healthy dinner staples.** On those nights when you didn't plan dinner, avoid takeout by keeping a few staples ready, such as pre-roasted chicken from the grocery store (these stay well in the freezer and can be quickly microwaved), precooked packets of rice and quinoa (dump into a microwave-safe bowl and nuke for ninety seconds), and frozen veggies (see hacks #3 and 5 to prep these in a flash). Dinner is good for everyone and ready in ten minutes.

- **Prevent unhealthy cravings in the first place.** Try to minimize temptations by keeping your body running on all four cylinders. Skipping meals or cutting sleep can both increase our cravings, while exercise can keep them in check.

Hack 21
Try Time-Restricted Eating

I have realized a couple of truths about myself: (1) I don't like counting calories, and (2) I like nutritional changes that don't make me feel like I'm missing out on anything. Which is why time-restricted eating (TRE) was my mainstay for losing fifty pounds of pregnancy weight after having my second child. You may have heard of intermittent fasting, a practice that many experts tout for weight loss and overall longevity benefits. TRE is like its younger, more laid-back sibling.

Here's how it works. You restrict the time window in which you eat, allowing for a "mini-fast" of twelve to sixteen hours daily during the night (say, from 8 P.M. to 8 A.M.). Because the mini-fast occurs largely while you're sleeping, you don't feel deprived. In a study where TRE participants were *not* told to reduce calories or make any dietary changes, participants lost 4 percent of their body weight in four weeks, slept better, and were more alert during the day.[6] TRE has also been linked to lower cholesterol and lower inflammation levels, and it has even been associated with a lower risk of breast cancer.[7] In a study in mice (because, well . . . science), those mice allowed to eat on a twenty-four- or fifteen-hour cycle became obese with increased inflammation, while those on the nine- or twelve-hour TRE schedule (who ate the exact same number of calories) lost weight, improved their insulin sensitivity, and reduced inflammatory markers—*even when they were allowed to cheat a little on weekends.*

Why does it work? For one, our bodies are designed to eat and sleep according to our circadian rhythm (CR), and our modern lives have disrupted that balance, making weight loss hugely difficult (read more on the circadian rhythm in the Sleep section starting on page 129). TRE-timed eating syncs our eating and CR, keeps us from eating in the late evening when we tend to eat mindlessly, and improves our sleep—all of which help naturally with weight loss.

- **Aim for either the nine- or twelve-hour eating window.** Choosing the nine-hour means you'd eat from 10 A.M. to 7 P.M., for instance; the twelve-hour could be 8 A.M. to 8 P.M. During the eating window, you just eat like you would normally: aim for a nutritious diet, but don't otherwise restrict (which is why I love it). Outside the eating window, stick to water or other non-calorie liquids.

- **It's okay to bounce back and forth between nine- and twelve-hour cycles.** In the mouse study, those in the nine-hour cycles lost the most weight and had the best health. But eating in a nine-hour window is really hard—especially with kiddos. So if there are days that you can make a nine- or ten-hour window work, pat yourself on the back. Otherwise, keep the window within twelve hours and call it a day.

- **Close the kitchen for your kids, too.** Tell everyone the kitchen closes at 9 P.M. (or earlier, depending on the age of your kiddos). Eating at all hours is bad for little mice—and little people as well.

- **It's okay to cheat!** I mean, if you weren't sold already, you will be now. The study on the mice found that those in the nine- or twelve-hour program remained lean, even if they cheated occasionally on weekends. Best news ever. Although that doesn't mean eat pizza at 2 A.M. every weekend, you can have a late dinner, snack, or drinks with friends without guilt.

Hack 22
Create Contingency Plans

Here, we steal a trick from smoking cessation programs. Just like eating, smoking has frequent "triggers" that can feel almost impossible to resist in the moment, despite your best intentions. So, when smokers aren't in the middle of a craving (and are able to think more clearly), we have them identify their triggers and find alternatives. That way, when the moment hits, they don't have to think—they can just enact their plan.

You can do the same. When you're not having a craving, identify your triggers to eat, and, choose a nonfood alternative for the next time the trigger strikes. In her book *Secrets from the Eating Lab,* leading food researcher Dr. Traci Mann says that contingency plans (see sample worksheet) work because (1) you come up with solutions when you're rational and not in the throes of a craving, and (2) instead of focusing on what you *can't* do, they focus on the new behavior that you *will* be doing.

- **Step 1.** Identify your biggest two or three overeating triggers.

- **Step 2.** Create a single contingency plan for each trigger ("When X trigger occurs, I will do B activity/make B choice"). Be specific—don't leave any decisions for the actual moment, or your cravings-obsessed brain will find a way to worm out. Write down the plan and repeat it out loud to yourself several times.

Trigger	Potential Contingency Plans
Overeating while crashing in front of the TV at the end of the day	Make it harder to eat while you watch TV: knit, do your nails (cheesy chips stuck to wet nail polish isn't a great look). Instead of your normal junk food snack, grab a healthier alternative, such as sparkling water and small pieces of fruit (so you still have the hand-to-mouth action) such as grapes or berries. Find ways to relax other than TV, such as taking a bath.
Overeating at parties	Don't arrive hungry—eat some veggies and good fats ahead of time. Keep your hands busy, such as carrying a drink in one hand and a napkin in the other, making it impossible to also hold a plate full of snacks. Research shows that when you try a little bit of everything you're more likely to overeat. So, instead of sampling many foods, survey all of the options, and then choose just three or four that you'll eat until you feel satisfied. Stand as far away from the buffet as possible, with your back to it.

Trigger	Potential Contingency Plans
Eating while driving	Find other things to do on your drive, like calling friends or listening to those podcasts you've been wanting to hear. Sing with your kids if they're in the car, or if they're not, just enjoy listening to music other than the *Moana* soundtrack (of course, please feel free to sing whether or not your kids are in the car. I won't judge). Take all food out of your car. If you need to carry snacks for the munchkins, keep them in a bin in the trunk, so you can't snack on them while driving.
Fill in your own triggers:	*Fill in your own contingency plans:*

Hack 23
Portion Control Made Easy

I grew up with horses, and we always knew that one of the biggest dangers to our horses was themselves—if one of them got loose and into the grain, the horse would overeat to the point of colic, a potentially life-threatening condition.

We humans are no different: *we don't stop eating when we're full; we stop eating when the food in front of us runs out.*

External signals such as our plate size and portions play as big a role (if not more) as our appetite in dictating how much we eat. That explains why over the past fifty years, as our portion sizes have grown astronomically, so have our waistlines.

But, just as a larger portion will lead us to eat more, on the flip side, smaller ones can have just the opposite effect.

- **Use plate size strategically.** In studies where people are unknowingly served different portion sizes, the larger the portion, the more they ate.[8] This even holds true for adolescents. (Younger children still seem to have the ability to listen to their internal fullness signals—a trait we should encourage and emulate!) Serve dessert/indulgent foods on smaller plates and healthier foods on bigger ones. You'll likely see the biggest effect in the family members who are unaware of the plate size swap, but even those who are aware (like you) may notice a difference in how much you eat, simply because it's not right in front of you.

- **Buy junk/comfort foods in smaller servings.** When people are given a large chocolate bar, they will eat substantially more than when they're given the same total amount in several smaller individually wrapped portions.[9] Junk food and distracted eating both bypass our natural satiety mechanisms, making it even more important in these situations that you purchase and serve smaller portions.

- **Serve food from the kitchen counter, not at the table.**
Even if you use smaller plates, you can still game the system by getting seconds . . . or thirds. Curb that habit by serving food at the kitchen counter, not at the table. That way, having seconds requires getting up from the table and walking into the kitchen, which can be just enough of an obstacle to that little extra helping.

- **Pack leftovers before you sit down to eat.** Once everyone has served themselves for a first round, put away leftovers (at least for those foods that you find most irresistible). You'll be even less likely to go back for seconds if you have to go into the fridge, unpack it, and reheat it.

Hack 24
Improve Workday Meals

If you're feeling like Elaine from *Seinfeld* with office cake for every celebration from birthdays to retirement, you may work with a cake pusher. In fact, for most of us, the office is a nutritional trap of stress, fatigue, and break-room treats.

If you have to use willpower to avoid a tempting treat at work, you're stealing focus that you actually *need* for deadlines or meetings. Remember that Roy Baumeister's research showed that when participants had to use willpower to resist eating chocolate, they gave up on a difficult project in half the time immediately after. In other words, when you're fixated on trying not to eat a donut, your boss's instructions just sound like "Wah wah wah, donut, cream filling, wah wah wah" (at which point you're not likely to *lean in* to anything but the candy bowl).

- **Bring your lunch.** It takes a few minutes of planning, but you'll eat a healthier meal if you bring it yourself. This works like a contingency plan because you identified and packed a healthy option when you were rational (and not hungry), so that when you're ravenous at 1 P.M., you'll have something good to eat locked in. One error I see is people packing too little, so they're still hungry; pack a healthy, filling meal, complete with veggies (as much as you think you'll want, and then add a little more), a starch, legumes, lean protein, and good fats.

- **Change the food environment.** Tempted by endless candy bowls at work? Ask HR to swap those out for fruit, serve a healthy breakfast or lunch once a week, or simply limit the treats to a single remote area. Most companies are desperate to find ways to keep their employees healthy and reduce health-care costs, so they may jump at this suggestion.

- **Keep healthy snacks in your desk/work fridge.** The other day, I had conference calls back to back to back. I couldn't leave my office (yes, I was doing jumping jacks on mute in my office to remain focused). But I still had a real lunch: a huge bowl of black bean soup, some almonds, and two plums. No, someone didn't deliver it. Keep shelf-stable foods in your desk, such as cartons of black bean or lentil soup and single-serving packets of nuts, as well as extra virgin olive oil and a small jar of really good balsamic vinegar to brighten up a salad. If you have access to a fridge, stock it with a bag of fruit, baby carrots, and hummus (which also doubles as a sandwich spread or salad topping).

Hack 25
Eat Well While Dining Out

No one wants to cook every night. There are nights that even the best dinner hacks don't cut it and you don't have the energy or time to cook or do dishes. When you do go out, follow these tips to keep everyone's nutrition on track.

- **General dining out tips:**

  - Leave off sauces such as mayo, ranch dressing, gravy, or any other cream-based sauce.

  - Replace fries with a vegetable. (I'm sorry. But you knew that was coming.)

  - Select meats that are grilled, broiled, poached, sous vide, or roasted.

  - Ask the waiter to box up half of your meal before you even get it.

  - Always start with a salad or broth-based soup.

  - For salad dressing, request an olive oil–based (or olive oil and vinegar) dressing on the side, or ask them to just use a half portion of their normal dressing amount. Leave off croutons and cheese.

  - Request that the server not bring out any bread.

  - Sip sparkling water, club soda, unsweetened tea, or even hot tea (which forces you to drink it slowly, and I find causes me to eat slowly, as a result).

  - Ask for a side of extra (not fried, no butter) veggies with olive oil.

  - Remember, you're there to visit with your friends or family, not just for the food. Take time to put down the fork and enjoy the company and the moment.

- **Skip the kids' menu.** Why is it that even at the nicer restaurants, where parents are getting broiled fish and salads, the kids' menus are predominantly fried chicken fingers and pizza? I have nothing against these periodically, but not every time. Set aside the fried food–laden kids' menu, and instead order your children's meals from the regular menu (they can split it with a sibling or take the rest for leftovers). Let them drink water or milk; no need for juice unless it's a very special treat.

- **Watch the alcohol.** Aside from its own calories, alcohol lowers your inhibitions and causes you to eat more. Women, on average, should have one drink daily, tops, and drink water in between sips. Wine is inherently difficult to chug (at least that tends to be frowned upon in public), making it a better choice over a sugary mojito that you'll polish off before you realize it.

- **Watch fast food.** Studies have also linked frequent fast food eating in kids with higher rates of obesity[10] and up to 55 percent higher levels of endocrine-disrupting phthalates,[11] so limit fast food to less than once a week.

- **Don't allow your dinner company to add to your waistline.** If your friend gains weight, you have a 170 percent higher chance of doing the same,[12] because our dining companions influence what we eat. It's okay to indulge every so often as a group, but if you consistently overeat with a particular friend, find nonfood activities to do together.

Getting the Whole Family Eating Well

Hack 26
Super-Hack Dinner

Eating at home is associated with lower weight and a better diet[1] (so your waist stays lean and your wallet fat). Plus, children who eat home-cooked meals more frequently have a healthier weight, and those who are involved in the cooking process consume more vegetables.[2]

Preparing a meal from scratch at home may sound daunting, but here's the secret: It rarely has to be *entirely* from scratch. You needn't slave all day over a hot stove (my grandmother used the phrase, and it sounds dramatic). With a combination of leftovers (or what I call the dinner miracle that keeps on giving) and other tips, preparing a meal at home takes only about ten minutes longer than takeout.

- **If you're not cooking enough protein for leftovers, you're not cooking enough.** Particularly when it comes to protein (which tends to be the most time-consuming portion of the meal), my philosophy is "cook once, eat twice." Roast two chickens for dinner tonight, then shred the remainders tomorrow for soup or pasta. Have fajitas tonight and use the leftover meat for chili tomorrow. (Sauté olive oil, garlic, and chili powder with a little tomato paste, tomatoes, beans, onions, corn, and beef broth and a bay leaf. Once your veggies are cooked, add the beef until hot.) Broil salmon tonight and add the leftovers to a veggie stir-fry tomorrow.

- **Don't have time to cook rice?** Packets are now available for brown rice, quinoa, and other grains and can be heated in the microwave for 90 seconds. Just pour them in a glass bowl to heat.

- **Double your veggies.** Whatever vegetable you're cooking tonight, double your recipe. Use leftovers for the next day's lunch as a salad or sandwich topping or repurpose it as a side for the next night's dinner. Steamed veggies one night can easily be tossed into a stir-fry, pasta, or soup the next night.

- **Ask your grocery meat department to prep the meat.** Whatever you're cooking, ask the meat department to cut the meat into the correct size that you'll need to cook (i.e., have them chop the chicken into stir-fry size, or the salmon or pork into kebab size), so that you won't have to chop. Don't be shy; the guy behind the meat counter at your grocery store can do this while you do the rest of your shopping. That simple request saves you time and raw meat handling (not to mention cleanup).

Hack 27
Easy Ways to Make Family Dinners Happen

Family time—it's what's for dinner.

Eating dinner together as a family isn't just a nicety; in fact, it's linked with kids eating more fruits, vegetables, calcium, and whole grains;[3] less binge eating;[4] and lowered risk of obesity.[5] Family dinner also boosts a child's psychosocial health and school performance,[6] while also reducing risky behaviors. Plus, it even enhances family communication and connectedness[7] and parents' health.[8] Yes, please.

But, with our overpacked schedules, regular family sit-down dinner can seem impossible. That's why there's great news: Dr. Jerica Berge (who clearly wants to help a mama out), an associate professor at the University of Minnesota Medical School, has studied family meals to identify what's really necessary (and what's not) to get the biggest bang for your buck.[9] Or, as Dr. Berge told me, she studies "what's the minimum amount of work you can do to get the family meal benefit?"[10]

- **Aim for a minimum of one or two family meals a week.** The more you eat together the better, but studies show that benefits start at even one to two shared meals a week. So if you're not doing family dinner at all, start there.

- **They can be short, but not too short.** This isn't Thanksgiving dinner. Aim for a meal that lasts approximately twenty minutes.

- **Eat in the kitchen or dining room with TV and devices off.** Kids who eat dinner without TV or devices are more likely to maintain healthy weight.[11] Not only is it distracting, the frequency of candy commercials has doubled since 2007,[12] making healthy eating even harder.

- **It's okay if both parents can't be there.** Research shows that having one *family-related adult* is necessary for "family dinner." But it needn't be *both parents* to get the beneficial effect if that's not possible.[13]

- **Add a vegetable.** It's okay if you didn't cook the meal from scratch. Even if you do takeout one night, Dr. Berge's research shows that just adding one home-prepped vegetable is associated with better health for everyone. Add a salad to takeout, microwave frozen veggies with olive oil, or serve raw veggies dipped in hummus.

- **Set dinner table standards and follow them.** What is it about dinnertime and a toddler that can turn even the sanest parents into either food dictators or pushovers? The best attitude is a middle-of-the-road style where parents are considerate of a child's preferences but keep standards for dinner behaviors.[14] That includes (1) allowing your child to give input into what is prepared, (2) cooking the same meal for everyone, and (3) having everyone sit down together at the same time.

- **Do not make a separate meal for a picky child.** It's one thing if your child likes the crust cut off his sandwich or the pepperoni taken off his pizza. But it's another if you're cooking a separate meal for him. Include one food that you know even your pickiest child will eat, but otherwise *do not cater to him.* Each individual may choose how much he eats (no forced "clean-plate club"), but everyone gets the same meal, *period.*

- **Encourage positive conversation.** We don't want any *For Keeps*–style "I'm pregnant. Can you pass the turnips?" at dinner. I'd suggest something a little lighter. If your questions are met with a single syllable "fine," consider a conversation starter like "roses and thorns" where everyone mentions one challenge they faced that day (thorn), and one thing for which they're grateful (rose).

Hack 28
Involve Your Kids in
Shopping/Prepping/Cooking

When I take my fifteen-month-old son to the grocery store, he smiles at all the women and gives them a "come hither" gesture (apparently that's the only way he knows how to wave), while making kissing noises. (*Now I know what it's like to go to the grocery store with Enrique Iglesias.*)

Although it may take longer, research shows that engaging your kiddos in meal planning, shopping, or prep increases the likelihood that they'll be open to—and eat—what's for dinner.

- **Let them have a voice in what you eat.** Get their input on family meals for the week. Give options such as "do you want salmon or chicken this week?" so you don't get suggestions of "ice cream!" for dinner. If you're cooking for that night, it can be as simple as "do you want rice or pasta tonight?" or "do you want carrots or green beans?"

- **Take them shopping.** Treat the produce section as a fun place to explore and discover. Allow a toddler to choose the apples or help you bag the peppers. Point out the colors of the grapes to a baby. For older children, take a moment to discuss a food label with them, marveling at the many unpronounceable ingredients in some processed foods. Go to your local farmers' market if you want to make food shopping even more of an experience, or take your kiddos to a local farm for fun and to see where their food really originates.

- **Give them adult versions.** Typically, some of the unhealthiest versions of foods are those that are manufactured for children. (Does that strike anyone else as heinous?) In one Yale University study, cereals targeted at children had 85 percent more sugar, 65 percent less fiber, 60 percent more sodium, and more artificial food coloring than typical "adult" cereals.[15]

- **Have your kids prep/cook dinner with you.** When kids participate in meal prep, they're more likely to feel positively about the meal and more in control.[16] They also eat more salad (76 percent more!) and lean protein.[17] Keep younger kids away from the stove and sharp items, but have them stir food, mix a salad, or set the table. My toddler loves getting messy while mixing chopped vegetables in olive oil and garlic, breaking ends off asparagus or green beans, and eating something she prepared.

- **Consider growing it yourself.** Children are more likely to taste[18] and eat more of produce that they helped grow.[19] No, you don't need Martha Stewart's or Ina Garten's farm; we have a small garden in the corner of our backyard in metro Atlanta, and even raised garden boxes on a patio or windowsill will work. Ask your local garden store what grows well in your area: I have good luck with tomatoes, peppers, squash, beans, and eggplant, but no matter what, I can't grow melon to save my life. Start small, experiment, and have fun together.

Hack 29
Offer Variety—and Don't Give Up

My daughter came home the other day and pointedly let me know that "Annie's mommy doesn't pack her fruit or vegetables for snack, she just gets to eat popcorn." Her preference was clear (thanks a million, Annie's mommy). *But part of the joy of adulting is that you don't have to be peer pressured by a four-year-old.* Take her preferences into account (which is why I'm happy to send popcorn), but you set the rules (such as expecting that she will eat the fruit and veggies along with it without fuss).

Most children inherently prefer sweet foods because their first food (breastmilk or formula) is sweet. Plus, "food neophobia," or an aversion to new flavors, was an instinct necessary for survival for our ancestor toddlers. Because our ancestors were toddlers, too, once.

So, when your toddler does her best Susan Lucci death-gag after eating a piece of zucchini, at least you now know why.

That doesn't mean it can't be overcome. You had this once, too—remember the first time you tried wine? I bet you didn't like it. *And now, look how far you've come.* During the so-called flavor window before eighteen months, tastes are particularly malleable, representing a great opportunity to introduce new flavors. However, even well beyond that age, you can still modify your child's taste preferences with a little persistence (just like you did for wine).

- **Expose your child to a wide variety.** Frequent exposure to a variety of whole foods increases a child's preferences for those foods years later.[20] Also, exposing your child to a broad array of flavors seems to prime her to be more adventurous with new flavors overall. One study showed that children who were given vegetable purees (peas, carrots) regularly for two weeks were more likely to eat an unfamiliar vegetable at the end of the study (artichoke puree in this study), so branch out beyond the rice cereal and milk/formula.[21] Start this as soon as your child is old enough to have purees.

- **Try to offer adventurous foods before he's gotten to the hangry point.** You want baby to be hungry, not so hungry that he's mad or crying.

- **Repetition, Repetition, Repetition.** It can be disheartening to cook a veggie and then have your child refuse it, which is why 90 percent of parents give up on a particular vegetable after offering it three to five times.[22] But that's too early; it can take up to ten introductions before some children accept a new food.[23] That means that the difference between your child liking and not liking a vegetable may simply be repetition (and patience—and wine). In one study, mothers were instructed to alternate a liked and a disliked veggie on separate days; by the end of two weeks, 70 percent of the children were eating the disliked vegetable as much as the liked one.

- **Leverage foods that they already like.** To further increase exposure to a variety of foods, leverage what foods they already enjoy. Like green peppers? Try red or orange. Vary flavors (such as green beans roasted with garlic and salt one night, then another veggie mixed into pesto and pasta with a little parmesan the next). If your child won't eat raw broccoli, cook it in teriyaki stir-fry. Try smoothies made with whole fruit (not juice) for a child reticent to eat fruit. Leverage hummus, salad dressing, or a dip your child likes to flavor an otherwise unfamiliar veggie.

- **"Eat your rainbow."** Turn produce eating into a contest by challenging your kids to eat as many colors in a day as possible. Think black grapes, purple cabbage, orange peppers, or pink papaya. And, no, rainbow-colored goldfish crackers don't count.

- **Snack time is a great chance to give fruits and veggies.** Snacks provide a great opportunity for extra produce when your child is hungry yet not distracted by an entire dinner. For infants, think very small pieces of strawberries, avocado, or cooked vegetables, and for toddlers give carrot sticks, chopped peppers, or broccoli with a bean dip, or grapes, apples, or melon. If your child is still hungry after eating the above, add some nuts, whole grain crackers, or cheese.

- **Adopt a "produce-first" philosophy.** Dr. Traci Mann refers to this as "be alone with a vegetable"; serving produce alone as an appetizer before each meal significantly increases the amount of fruits and veggies eaten.[24] Breakfast? Put out a bowl of berries. Lunch or dinner? Start with a salad, or cut up carrots and peppers and serve with hummus. These buy you time while you're preparing the meal and leverage your child's appetite to overcome food resistance. We do this every night for dinner—and even if dinner is actually ready, I'll stall and pretend that it's still cooking (you guys, don't tell my kids, please), to ensure they have time to eat veggies.

Hack 30
Adjust Your Food-Parenting Behavior

As a parent, you have a major impact on your child's lifetime taste preferences and weight.[25] But kids can be tricky, often influenced by your unconscious behavior or taking your example in the opposite way you intended. That's particularly so when it comes to language that's judgmental, coercive, and even in the case of (let's be honest and admit that we all do it) begging and negotiating. As good as our intentions may be, or how well these behaviors may seem to work in the short term, they backfire in the end. Follow these tips to make sure that your frame of mind sets the scene for good habits.

- **Avoid making certain foods entirely off limits.** It's like the boy that your parents told you to never date: The more forbidden something is, the more appealing it can seem. Consider letting your child have a certain food occasionally when you go out to eat but just not keeping it at home. That way, a food isn't forbidden, it's just not readily available.

- **Find non-health benefits for the foods.** Just like the lite label does for you, calling a food healthy can backfire. In one study, labeling a drink healthy caused children to rate it less enjoyable and less likely to ask their parents to buy it.[26] Instead, talk about other benefits. My daughter wants a unicorn for her birthday (yeah . . . *you* tell her . . .), so we call her salad "unicorn food." Grapes and edamame can be fun to eat because they "explode" in your mouth. Slightly older children would understand and appreciate "this food will help you have more energy at soccer" or "increase your focus in class."

- **Don't make unhealthy foods the reward for the healthy.** It can be tempting to say, "no dessert until you eat your veggies," but it will backfire in the long run. Using food as any sort of reward teaches children that the unhealthy foods are the yummy rewards and that the healthy ones are something to force down.

- **Don't create a comfort food connection for your child.** Many of us developed the comfort food connection as chil dren, where a stressful day meant that we needed a bowl of ice cream. Your child is a clean slate. Prevent this habit from even developing by showing them that if something's bothering them, they can find non-food solutions: turn on music and dance. Run. Play. Share a challenge with you to problem-solve together or write in their journal. Showing them that they can find solutions outside the kitchen isn't just good for their waistlines—it's empowering.

- **Keep the food judgment to a minimum.** Instead of lectures such as "There are starving children in the world and you're wasting food" (Didn't work when your mom said it. Still doesn't.), turn the food discussion into one of curiosity. Ask, "Where do you think this was grown?" or find descriptive statements such as "Eating this makes my bones grow stronger."

- **Remember that little eyes are watching what you eat.** Research is clear that children tend to eat what their parents eat.[27] Which is why although I like salt, seeing my daughter start reaching for the salt shaker has led us to switch to a salt-free mix of herbs. Similarly, watch your own reaction to a new food: you can't expect your child to eat it if you or your partner wrinkles their nose with every bite.

Hack 31
Troubleshoot Picky Behavior

My son, who is my second child, will eat anything that doesn't eat him first. My daughter, however, is a little more . . . well . . . *independent.* She'll eat green beans today but not tomorrow. Or she'll ignore the stir-fry vegetables and chicken I cooked and only eat quinoa. I try not to take it to heart. The reality is that, at any point in time, up to 20 percent of parents would characterize their children as picky eaters.[28]

"Picky eating" can range from mild avoidance (like with my daughter) to refusing to touch a particular food group. The good news is that 60 percent of kids labeled picky will outgrow it within two years.[29] Unless your child has a health problem that prevents him from eating a wide variety of foods, you can change his eating habits.

- **Sanity saver 1: Stop stressing about it. Your child will not starve.** Your job is not to make sure your child swallows the food. Your job is to keep offering it and to model eating it yourself. It's the child's decision whether to eat it.

- **Sanity saver 2: They don't have to eat every food group at every meal.** Aim for a balanced *week*; it's okay if he doesn't hit every food group in a single meal—or *day*. Some days he may eat everything at breakfast, then just protein for lunch, and veggies at dinner. With your pediatrician's blessing, don't make yourself crazy about having three square meals.

- **Give options.** Pull a few tricks from Game Theory (a model from economics to influence behavior) and allow your child to feel in control. Instead of just putting two foods on your child's plate and expecting him to eat both, put three or four healthy options (think a protein, a starch, and a vegetable or two), and allow him to choose which ones he eats. He feels like he has "won" by choosing what he eats, and you win because he ate healthy food.

- **Stand your ground.** When you can (and especially when you're home and your child's protests can't bother anyone else), stand firm. The meal is what's offered, and no number of tantrums will change that. Make it clear that dinner is the food for the night, and that grabbing something from the pantry is not an option. Unless your pediatrician is concerned about your child's weight and growth, she will survive skipping dinner that night. Sure, her protesting makes dinner more stressful for everyone, but it won't last forever, and the more consistent you are, the sooner it will end. Breathe.

- **Consider inviting one of his friends who eats well to join you.** There's nothing wrong with using a little peer pressure for a good cause. If your child has a friend who you've noticed eats fruits and veggies readily, have them eat together. Just like how your friends eat influences *you*, it will also do so for your child.

- **Stop buying the unhealthy options.** If eating junk food starts to become a huge battle with your child, just stop buying it. You hold the credit card (*adulting has its perks*). Although they may protest at first, most young children will forget about it after one or two weeks. On the flip side, make sure that many healthy options are available to fill in the gap left by the absent snacks.

PART 2
Exercise

The Basics

Finding Time

Making It Fun

Finding the Motivation and Building the Habit

When the Going Gets Hard

C hris Norton was someone else who was told "never." When he was nineteen, a bad tackle left him paralyzed from the neck down, and he was told the words no one ever wants to hear, that he "would never walk again."[1]

He didn't listen, either.

In 2018, seven years after his injury, he walked his bride seven yards down the aisle. But, for him, those steps meant so much more. He said, "This walk isn't about the physical act of walking[,] it is about not letting your challenges and setbacks keep you down."[2]

Sometimes, exercise is so pushed as a thing we "have to do" that we forget the sheer magic of what we can do with our feet and arms and body. And we didn't always feel this way. In fact, there was a time when we all loved physical activity. We called it recess, and, for most of us, it was probably our favorite class (a close second to snack time).

Our bodies were made to move. It feels good—like laughing. But, somewhere along the way growing up, we seem to have unlearned a few things, such as how to snort milk out our noses, how to rock striped leggings with polka dot socks and a paisley dress without self-consciousness, and how good it feels to just *play*.

At some point, recess became exercise, which became "no pain, no gain" workouts, which . . . well . . . just became *work*— and something we started to dread.

After gaining forty-five pounds with my first child, I wasn't exactly comfortable in my postpartum body. So, as soon as I got the medical all clear, because I didn't have any fancy Hollywood trainers at my beck and call, I put my baby in the stroller and hustled out the door on a walk. I'd never been much of a walker—it seemed too *easy*. But, post-baby, I started to think differently: I realized my postpartum shape wasn't some debt for which I had to be penalized. Exercise didn't have to punish my body. In fact, walking was one of the best ways I could *love* my shape. For the first time in years, I realized that I *didn't need to suffer to get the benefits of physical activity.*

Exercise can feel *good*. And if the first thing you try doesn't feel good, find something else.

Not only does exercise give you direct health benefits, it also unlocks benefits everywhere else in your life (see more in hack #32). Exercise is my survival tool, my get-through-the-day, only-way-I-can-get-everything-done-and-stay-sane tool. Of course, that doesn't mean that it's always easy to fit it in or that you'll always *want* to do it, which is why you have this chapter.

Two weeks after one of my friends implemented a few hacks from this chapter, her nine-year-old cautiously asked her, "You're in such a good mood lately . . . why?" My desire for you is that by the end of this chapter, you have some habit of movement. I don't care how small it is—simply that you can sustain it and that makes you feel *good*.

It's time to remember the joy of movement, and, as Richard Simmons told us, it's time to "move those buns." Are you ready?

The Basics

Hack 32
Find Your "Why" for Exercise

Chris Norton spent hours in the gym for his wedding—but it wasn't so he'd fit into his tux. It was because he wanted to walk his bride down the aisle. In fact, he has posted on Instagram, "Grinding to be able to walk @emilysummers08 7 yards down the aisle after we get married. . . . 7 years of hard work is going into this one moment and it will be so worth it!"[1] Exercise for him had a true purpose and meaning. When he was tired or didn't feel like it—as every one of us all feels at times—it was that purpose that made it all worthwhile.

Which is why, just like I had you do for nutrition, I'll ask you to find your "why" for exercise. Of course, there are the direct health benefits, and starting an exercise habit to fit into your pre-pregnancy jeans can be a kick start, but research shows that having a more intrinsic motivation substantially increases your chance of success.[2] If your only reason for going for a walk is to lose a few pounds, dropping today's walk may not seem like such a big deal. But if you consider your "why"—that not walking today will make you more stressed and more likely to snap at your child, to sleep more poorly, or to have less energy for your side-hustle, taking that walk is suddenly endowed with much greater meaning—you're more likely to do it.

Exercise has far more benefits than just the physical; when people start exercising—even without intending to make other changes—they naturally discover downstream benefits. They sleep better, their personal interactions are better, and they even subconsciously start to eat better and give up bad habits such as smoking.

Kyle and Brent Pease are brothers who compete in Ironman races. In fact, they complete every race together. You see, Kyle has cerebral palsy and is unable to use his arms and legs, so Brent and Kyle complete their races together as a team, with the use of a special kayak, custom bicycle, and racing wheelchair. Brent may be the one running, but he says that he couldn't do the races without Kyle, telling us that "Kyle borrows my legs, but I borrow his spirit." It's Kyle who keeps them going, through even the darkest, longest miles, and they've created the Kyle Pease Foundation to share the joy of sports with others with disabilities.

Kyle Pease and Chris Norton are both proof that it's not your physical capacity but your meaning—your heart—that propels you forward.

You've got the legs—what gives you *your* heart? Choose a meaningful reason from the list below or find your own.

- **You'll live longer.** Regular exercise is one of the best things we can do to extend our life span, cutting risk of death by 40 percent. It lowers your risk for chronic disease and cancer and keeps you vibrant longer, combatting the annual bone and muscle loss that starts in middle age.[3]

- **You're more productive and your brain functions better.** Too busy to exercise? You're too busy not to. Exercising for thirty minutes three times a week increases mental

performance by 15 percent and yields immediate benefits
for creativity, executive functioning, and memory. It cuts
your risk of dementia by a factor of ten.[4] My running
breaks maintained my sanity while I was writing this
book—and gave me bolts of inspiration when I was stuck
with writer's block.

- **It makes you happier.** "Exercise gives you endorphins.
Endorphins make you happy. Happy people don't kill their
husbands. They just don't."[5] Sure, Elle Woods said it, but
so did Duke University. In a study of major depression,
Duke researchers found that regular exercise was as beneficial as taking an antidepressant,[6] except without the side
effects. Exercise also acts through your endocannabinoid
receptors (yes, the same receptors activated by marijuana)
to lower stress, anxiety, and to better regulate anger.[7]

- **You'll sleep better.** Whether you have true insomnia or
just a little mom-somnia and hypervigilance, exercise helps
you fall asleep sooner and sleep better.

- **You'll have more energy.** One study showed that just
twenty minutes of exercise three times a week led to 20
percent more energy and 65 percent less fatigue.[8]

- **It gives you more willpower.** You've heard me say that
willpower is a finite resource; we drain away at it all day
long. Regular exercise works as willpower training, boosting your willpower store every day and making other
healthy decisions easier.

- **It's important for your kids.** Exercising early in life and
often impacts a child's health (of course), but also development, behavior, and even gut microbiome (our belly bugs
need their cardio, too). Exercise also provides a great opportunity to spend time together: as your children grow up,

an active tradition such as a weekly hike or family kickball game preserves precious family time.

- **Because you'll eat better.** Research shows that people who exercise also tend to eat better, even if that was not their original goal.[9]

- **Because it's *fun*.** Choose the right exercises, the right music, and the right workout buddies, and exercise can be fun again.

- **What are *your* reasons?** Feel free to use any of the above, or make up your own.

- _____
  _____

- _____
  _____

- _____
  _____

Hack 33
What's Recommended and Where to Start

Before we get creative in hacking your exercise, let's start with what's recommended. The American Heart Association recommends 150 minutes a week of moderate cardio *or* 75 minutes of vigorous-intensity cardio, plus 30 minutes per week of strength training. That may sound daunting, so remember that you don't need to accomplish all of it today—it's a *goal*, and we absolutely give partial credit!

Baby Exercise Steps

If you haven't exercised in a while, start slowly. Aim for just one exercise session a week, or just ten minutes a day. Start where you are, do what you can, and proceed with baby steps so that you can feel success by meeting attainable goals. Otherwise, if you set unrealistic expectations, the disappointment of failing to reach impractical goals can derail you before you even start.

What to Do   Amount

CARDIO	**75–150 minutes weekly:** If you do only moderate intensity, aim for 150; if you add some vigorous activity, aim for 75–150.

Moderate intensity: You should be able to talk. Heart rate should be around 50–70 percent, or around 90–126 bpm (beats per minute) for the average forty-year-old.

Brisk (not speed) walking

Doubles tennis

Ballroom dancing (hey, you wanted suggestions)

Gardening

Bicycling < 10 mph

Vigorous intensity: You can say a few words, but not a full sentence. Heart rate 70–85 percent, or around 125–155 bpm for the average forty-year old.

Speed walking

Jogging

Running

Swimming laps

Bicycle > 10 mph

Jumping rope

STRENGTH TRAINING	30 minutes/week

You can accomplish this using real weights or exercises that use your body as weight.

MOM HACK RECOMMENDATION:
Combine Cardio and Strength into One Workout

When time is tight, combine cardio *and* strength together, like some of the more intense workouts below.

Hiking/walking with your child in a carrier

Pushing your child in a stroller while jogging (especially on hills)

Boot-camp/cross-training workouts

Jogging combined with intervals of sprints or pushups and mountain climbers

Hill sprints (jogging somewhere hilly and sprinting uphill[10])

My 10-Minute High Intensity Workout:
- Jog in place/jump rope in place for 3 minutes to warm up
- Then do each exercise for 30 seconds:
  Squats
  Pushups
  Lunges
  Plank
  Burpees
  Triceps dips
  Jumping jacks
  Mountain climbers
  One-arm row (with a weight)
  Scissor kicks
- Jog in place/jump rope in place for 2 minutes, then repeat routine two or three times, or as time allows

Hack 34
Get the Whole Family Exercising

When my house gets particularly chaotic, you'll hear me say, "Everyone outside *now*." Keeping my kiddos active is as important for my *sanity* as it is for their *health*.

According to the Centers for Disease Control and Prevention, children today get much less activity than we did as kids: less than 25 percent of children get the recommended sixty minutes of physical activity per day.[11] Not only does exercise lower kids' risk of obesity, it improves reading, math, and classroom behavior.[12]

Create a habit of being active as a family, and it quickly becomes self-sustaining. Plus, our partners influence our likelihood of exercising by as much as 40 percent; if one doesn't exercise, the other is more likely to give it up. But if you both exercise, you'll each reinforce the other's habit, and partners who exercise together report greater relationship satisfaction, more feelings of love,[13] and do more *you-know-what*.

- **Exercise together as a family, and don't overthink it.** You don't need some formal workout. In a study of parents, simply finding ways to be physically active with their kids, like bringing baby along on a hike, was effective,[14] even for parents who hadn't exercised in a while.[15] Simply send everyone outside to run around, and they will play.

- **Join your child's play activity.** Instead of sitting on the sideline in the park or backyard, join your child. (If you haven't tried monkey bars since you were eleven, prepare for a shock. They got *much* harder.) Play tag, soccer, or catch, or have a jump-rope contest. Join them at the indoor play zone or in the local pool. Not only will you get exercise, but also fun quality time together, which your kids will appreciate. (Until they turn twelve, at which point they'll pretend they don't know you.)

- **Make regular activity a family norm.** With screens and their billions of toys (the next person who gives my child a toy that beeps is taking my child *home* with them), sometimes it takes coaxing to put down the devices and be active. Make daily activity a family norm, and it will be questioned less. We have a rule of "thirty minutes outside play before dinner." We go outside (raincoats if it rains, as long as there's no lightning), or otherwise play hide and seek or dance inside. You can also start new family traditions, such as a weekly Saturday hike, or a Wednesday night backyard kickball.

- **Dance together at night.** One of my favorite family activities is a family dance party. Let everyone take turns choosing the music so that it's fun for everyone; our current favorite is Brandon Flowers's "Magdalena." (And no, none of us have any idea what the lyrics mean, but it's better than listening to "Let It Go" again.)

- **Go for a walk together.** Depending on your child's age, put him in the baby carrier, stroller, or allow him to walk, and head out (when she was younger, my daughter would ride in the stroller for a bit, walk a bit, and then ride again when she got tired).

- **Get pedometers for everyone in your family.** Competitive much? Then get everyone pedometers. Compete with each other, with your siblings and their families for most steps, or in a parents versus kids contest. Or, just as a family, aim for a single goal such as 8,000 steps per person over age six. When that's achieved, reward everyone with something like a day at the park together or a trip to the zoo.

- **Use your "baby weight."** Make baby your weights to get exercise—and giggles. Do squats while baby's in the carrier, bicep curls, shoulder raises, or chest presses, each time using baby as your adorable weight. For older children, give them a piggy back ride on an afternoon walk or carry a toddler in your arms for some bonding time and serious upper body workout.

- **Activities by age for your child:**

  - **Infants:** Give baby ample tummy time and let her strengthen her arms by gripping your fingers. Encourage kicks and reaching by laying her on a mat with toys hanging overhead, or on one that plays a tone when she kicks a keyboard.

  - **Toddlers:** Activity at this age can be pretty basic: throwing, kicking, running. Kick or roll a ball back and forth, ride a tricycle, or walk on a line. Play a game of tag, follow the leader, or ring around the rosy. Jump over (or through) the sprinkler.

  - **Preschoolers and older:** Incorporate balance activities (such as balancing on one foot, hopping, or hopscotch in the driveway), somersaults (another activity that seems to have gotten harder as I got older) and other gymnastics, swimming, and riding tricycles or bicycles with training wheels. Games with instructions, such as Simon Says, duck-duck-goose, or red light/green light are fun at this age, as is hide-and-seek. Children this age may even enjoy doing an exercise video with you, and older children can start to join you on a short jog.

Hack 35
Increase Your Daily Activity, Period

Research is clear—sitting for more than 25 percent of your day is bad for you. So, make it a daily habit to just *move* whenever you can. If your butt starts to take on the waffle indentations of your chair, you've been sitting too long. By incorporating even the smallest opportunities, before you know it, you've accumulated a day's worth of steps.

In fact, in a study where women were assigned to either (A) a group told that they had to get their physical activity through a daily structured aerobic exercise program or (B) a group instructed to just get more general movement into their lives (such as walking short distances instead of driving or taking the stairs), those in group B lost more weight and kept it off.[16] That's not to say that you shouldn't work out—but sometimes the simplest ways are the best.

- **Fidget.** Stuck in a meeting or on a plane? Fidgeting can counteract the effects of prolonged sitting.[17] Change your position every few minutes or alternate straightening and bending your knees. Or, silently tap your toes under the table: researchers at the University of Missouri showed benefits from tapping your foot for one minute, resting it for four minutes, and repeating the cycle.

- **Stand up.** Stand up when you're on a work call or webinar (especially if they can't see you). It may even help you focus better[18] and sound more engaged. If I'm the only one in my office on a miserably long call, I'll walk back and forth behind my desk or even do jumping jacks (on mute). (Yes, I have a coworker who sees me do this through my office window. Yes, he laughs. I care not.) Take walk breaks when you've hit a mental wall or a "walking meeting" or "walking phone call" when possible. If you have a wearable device that encourages you to stand up every hour, that's a fantastic reminder to stand.

- **Any time you can choose the active choice, take it.** I have a coworker who will only use the bathroom on different floors from her office, forcing herself to take the stairs every bathroom break, and I think it's genius. Drink water at your desk so that you're getting up for regular bathroom breaks (and refill your water bottle each time). If you take public transportation, get off the subway or the bus a stop or two early and walk the distance. Or if you drive, park a little farther away and walk in. Choose stairs over the elevator. Walk to lunch or to drop off the letter at the post office. Or . . . (gasp) *walk* to your colleague's desk, instead of texting or sending an e-mail. (I know. It sounds like an extreme sport, doesn't it?)

- **Make your social events active.** Want to catch up with a girlfriend? Meet for a walk instead of a drink (or a walk, *then* a drink, if you're ambitious). Have your date night include a walk, bowling, or any physical activity.

- **Have a list of "burst" activities to do in downtime.** Waiting in carpool? Stuck on hold? TV on a commercial break? Have a list of two or three activities you can do for anywhere from one to five minutes.

Jumping jacks	Squats
Burpees	Wall-sits
Planks	Touch the ground,
Lunges	then jump in the air

- **Carry your baby on short trips.** Instead of putting your child in the stroller, for short trips carry him. You know that it takes longer to take the darn stroller out of the trunk, anyway.

Finding Time

Hack 36
Start with Fifteen Minutes a Day

A friend of mine told me that she had skipped exercising that morning because she didn't have a solid thirty minutes to exercise. *Hold up*—there are no exercise police who say that you only get "exercise credit" if you go for thirty minutes or more. You know what's worse than just doing a partial workout? Not exercising at all.

Truth #1: You *absolutely* can get a benefit from exercising—for whatever amount of time you have.

Truth #2: You're more likely to do a shorter workout. A study showed that people who aim for multiple, shorter bouts of exercise (like two 10-minute workouts a day) actually exercised more per week and lost more weight than those who exercised only when they had a single block of forty minutes.[1]

Plus, the shorter the time commitment, the easier it is to create an exercise habit (see hack #46 for more on creating habits).

- **Start with ten minutes a day.** If you exercise less than once a week, I ask you to give me ten minutes a day. All it takes is ten minutes to boost your mood. Really. Ten minutes of doing any activity that you want. If you already are doing ten minutes a day, add another five to ten minutes, as each incremental ten minutes will take you to the next level, health-wise.

- **If you can't give me ten minutes, start with five.** I'm serious. If your days are erratic, do five minutes of exercise as soon as you wake up. It's short enough that you can squeeze it into even the most chaotic days, to build an exercise habit.

- **Do multiple, shorter bouts.** Break a workout into multiple, shorter intervals on the days that you don't have a solid thirty-minute block (or when your motivation is low and thirty minutes seems sooooo long). On those days, do two fifteen-minute sessions, or even three ten-minute ones.

- **On short-bout days, up the intensity.** Not only does high intensity up your metabolism all day long, science shows that it may also improve your attention and focus. On your short-bout days, make at least one session high intensity.

Hack 37
Choose a Schedule That Fits You

Timing is everything. Not only does *when* you exercise influence your exercise adherence, it also affects how exercise feels, how you feel for the rest of the day, your circadian rhythm (CR), metabolism, and sleep.

Use this cheat sheet to identify the best exercise times for you.

If you have trouble falling asleep	4–5 P.M.	Your body temperature elevates during a workout, then drops after four or five hours. Exercise at 4–5 P.M. (see hack #38, to keep kiddos occupied), and that natural temperature drop coincides with a 10–11 P.M. bedtime, helping you fall asleep. But don't intensely exercise less than four hours before bed, or the energy burst from exercise may keep you awake. If that's the only time you can exercise, stick to something low intensity, such as Pilates or easy walking.
If you have trouble waking up in the morning	First thing in the morning	I know; it sounds counterintuitive. But a consistent morning workout can shift your CR forward, boosting your A.M. energy and making mornings easier.
To increase your chances of sticking to it	Morning	Mothers who stick to a fitness regimen are most likely to work out in the morning, before any of their work or mom duties get in the way.[2]
To be social with coworkers	At lunch	Have a coworker with similar health goals? Take a yoga class, walk, or a jog weekly together over lunch, and grab a quick meal after at your desk.

For better athletic performance	Afternoon / early evening	Our body temperature is higher in the afternoon, with faster reaction times and lower heart rate and blood pressure. That makes us stronger, we perform better, and we're less likely to be injured.
To burn fat	Morning	It takes about 20 minutes for your body to start burning fat as fuel during a workout. Make that happen more quickly by working out while your body is still "fasting" before breakfast.
To find what works for you	Experiment	For two weeks, workout twice a week in the morning. If you still find it hard, try another time, like late afternoon or early evening. When do you feel better, have more energy, and enjoy it more?

Hack 38
Squeeze in Exercise
When the Kids Want to Play

In a world where you can't even pee without an interruption, free time for exercise is rare, assuming that you can even get someone to watch your kids. When you can't sneak away, you have two options: (1) work out with them (hack #34) or (2) follow these sneaky tricks to buy yourself time. As Dr. Jerica Berge told me,

"Incorporate physical activity into time with your kids, because it's otherwise probably not going to happen on its own."[3]

- **Special toys for when mommy's exercising.** If you want to do a workout video or use home exercise equipment, set aside special toys that your children only get to play with while you exercise. Put the toys away when you're done exercising, so they retain the mystique and "fun" factor to keep their attention the next time.

- **Phone timer intervals.** If your child wants you to play with her, set your phone timer for five minutes and hand her the phone. Do a high intensity exercise (running on the treadmill, bicycle, or just jumping jacks and burpees) for five minutes, then play with her for five minutes. Repeat that cycle until you complete your workout. Yes, it takes longer, but your child is happy and feels in control, and the intervals can give you a killer workout.

- **Exercise at snack or naptime.** Make your exercise time their snack time, whether they're sitting in the stroller on a walk/jog or you're working out at home. Hand them their afternoon/morning snack, and you've bought at least a few minutes for an intense interval. Of course, naptime is a beautiful interval for you to get in a workout interruption-free. The laundry and full dishwasher can wait.

Hack 39
Use Gym-Free Options

There's no law that says you have to go to the gym to get exercise. In fact, I rarely go. My husband does regularly, but I can complete my run in a half-hour at home, without a commute, so it's a huge time-saver.

If you don't have a gym membership, don't have the time to get there, or just don't like it, that's entirely fine. Find non-gym options instead.

- **Get equipment at home.** One study showed that people who have exercise equipment at home are more likely to fit in exercise, lose weight, and maintain that weight loss.[4] It doesn't take much: a single piece of cardio equipment, a few hand weights, and you're good to go. Save money on costly equipment by checking the local used fitness equipment store or your Facebook local groups. Or use the money you'd otherwise spend on an unused gym membership on home equipment instead. Depending on your health insurance plan and general health, some insurers may even compensate you for the cost.

- **Use a DVD or YouTube exercise video.** Consider a workout video that requires only a few hand weights, if anything at all. All you need is a TV, laptop, or any device with Wi-Fi, and a little space.

- **Walk around your neighborhood.** Data from multiple studies show that people who simply walk at home are far more likely to stick to their walking program and increase their weight loss.[5]

- **Exercise outdoors.** Exercising outdoors leads to better energy, and even less anger and depression.[6] It also creates more variability than using a single piece of equipment. Fun science fact: Researchers have found that some fat cells *may* shrink in size when exposed to sunlight. There's more research to be done there (don't pull a Brandi Chastain while you're running to up your sun exposure *just yet*), but consider it another reason to head outside.

Hack 40
Discover Pockets of Time to Exercise

It feels like we can't squeeze another moment out of our busy days, but if you intentionally look for them, you'll find small pockets of time. Use even the smallest windows to exercise (five minutes works!), and you'll find that these short workouts accumulate over the course of the week. Just try to log your activity when you're doing short intervals, so you can see how far you've come—and congratulate yourself.

- **During your child's activities.** As one mom told me, the only time she can be active is during her kids' activities. If they're at soccer, she walks around the soccer fields. If they're at the gym, she'll walk the track.[7]

- **In the carpool line.** How much of our lives do we waste in a carpool line? (Don't answer that. It's the bane of parenting existence.) If time is short, do calf raises, squats, and other exercises by your car. *Who cares what the other parents think—some wish they had thought of it.* Got there early? Go for a walk/jog. Take any siblings in a stroller and give your cell number to the driver in line behind you (that is, if she doesn't join you).

- **Do a childcare swap with your partner or neighbor.** Trade childcare with your partner or a friend while the other exercises. Negotiate workout times with your partner: Say, one runs in the morning, and the other works out in the evening. You're helping each other be healthy and can even keep each other motivated.[8]

- **Turn off social media.** Honestly. Do you need to scroll through Facebook for thirty minutes every day? That's a full workout right there.

Making It Fun

Hack 41
Find Exercises That Match
Your Personality

I'm frequently asked, "What's *the* best exercise for me to lose weight?" Here's the thing—there's no one magic exercise for everyone. The *best* exercise isn't one that I prescribe for you—but the one you enjoy.

In fact, although *all* exercise boosts your mood and lowers anxiety, when you do an activity that you choose and prefer, endocannabinoid levels (chemicals that help our moods and regulate anger) are even higher.[1]

Research suggests your personality type may predict the exercise you'll stick to the best,[2] so choose the two or three personality features in the table below that best describe you, and try the matching activities. Keep experimenting. Exercise should make you feel good, feel invigorated. So, if one doesn't, try another. You may be surprised by what sticks!

Personality Feature	Defining Features	Good Activities
EXTROVERTED	Extroverted people feel more energy, motivation, and adherence when they workout with others. Extroverts are also more drawn to aerobic activities.[3]	Team sports Group training classes Dance Exercising with a buddy Working out in a gym where you can interact with others
INTROVERTED	Introverts stick to a workout longer if they're able to do it alone.	Swimming Running Cycling Working out at a gym while wearing headphones.
CONTROLLED	If you like to have control over when/how long you do things, choose an exercise that you can dictate.	Swimming Tai chi Weight training Running Yoga
COMPETITIVE	Choose activities that involve "winning" to motivate you to keep going. Sign up for a competition to up the stakes.	Team sports Racquet sports Group training Golf Running Swimming Cycling/spinning

Personality Feature	Defining Features	Good Activities
INTUITION-DRIVEN	People who rely heavily on intuition can get bored easily with exercise. They need variability, novelty or an adrenaline-filled experience.	Downhill or water skiing A pass/membership that gives you access to many different gyms and class types Dance Rock climbing If you run/walk, vary your routes Extreme sports (go, Mom!)
CREATIVE	People who like working with new ideas thrive in outdoor exercise settings.	Running Cycling Walking Hiking
LOGIC-DRIVEN	These exercisers adhere to programs longer that are based on evidence.	Choose a trainer/class based on the highest-qualified instructors you respect
FEELINGS-DRIVEN	These exercisers value a connection with their exercise partners.	Choose a trainer with whom you really connect, or work out with a friend

Hack 42
Make It Social

No mom is an island. Despite the fact that we are surrounded by munchkins all day, mom-ing can be a lonely task. Keep those connections by engaging a friend in your fitness plan, and you'll keep both your body and your friendship strong.

If you know someone is monitoring you or depending on you to exercise, you're far more likely to do it. In addition to making it more fun, friends can also put positive social pressure on each other, in which case your friend's healthy habits can rub off on you.

- **Work out together.** If you can get the timing to work, having an exercise buddy is fabulous for adherence—and can even boost how hard you exercise.[4] Go for a walk together, play tennis, or attend a fitness class. It's hard to find time with my girlfriends nowadays, and this is a great way to get exercise *and* girl time.

- **Track each other on an app.** Even if you can't work out together, leverage technology to keep each other honest. One girlfriend and I are linked on a fitness app. Every time I log my weight or fitness activity, she sees it, and vice versa. Knowing that the other is watching increases our accountability, plus we can also send each other little encouraging messages. Many fitness apps will now let you do this for free.

- **Compete against each other.** Many fitness apps will also let you join a challenge with friends, coworkers, your college roommates, or even other app users. Compete for steps, minutes exercised, miles, or any other metric to keep you moving forward.

Hack 43
Play Music to Motivate You

You may not know it, but Brit-Brit can actually help you complete your workout (I am pretty sure that she did *intend* to say, "You gotta work[*out*] b***ch"). Studies show that the right music can boost your endurance and performance, relax your blood vessels,[5] and even make the exercise seem 20 percent easier.[6] Remember Michael Phelps and his omnipresent headphones during the Olympics? It wasn't just because Beats look cool.

For me, I love running while listening to dance music from my young and carefree pre-kiddo years. *Which is why half the songs on my playlist are over ten years old. Except for "Despacito," because I obviously know "how they do it in Puerto Rico." (No, no I really don't.)*

- **Choose what you like.** What music motivates you is personal, which is why I always hated that gym class where the instructor played Grateful Dead. What worked for her, did *not* work for me. Michael Phelps reportedly listens to Eminem, Eric Church, and Young Jeezy. Olympic water polo player Maggie Stevens likes Andra Day's "Rise Up," while the Canadian track and field team gets psyched to Kanye. Maybe you like old-school Christina Aguilera or hair rock. I'm not going to judge. And if you're asking, I run to Bruce, Gaga, Sia, and Queen, among others. You can find my playlist at www.drdarria.com/momhacks (password: unstoppable), and we can listen together.

- **Choose the right tempo and intensity.** Choose music with a beats per minute, (BPM) that matches your exercise pace. For running, that usually means music with around 120–130 BPM (search online for songs with that speed).

Plus, many running or music apps can detect your running pace and select a playlist that matches.

- **Pregame.** If you can't listen to music while you're exercising, listen to it just before you work out to up your game.

Hack 44
Get Your Village Active

To truly change your and your family's health, engage your neighborhood and community. Research from Dr. Jerica Berge shows that getting your "village" engaged in physical activity even helps the adults with weight loss.[7] In fact, she demonstrated that it can also have a halo effect: Once people started doing activities as a group, they were more likely to also do them on their own. The healthier your community is, the healthier you and your family are.

- **Make neighborhood parties active.** The next time you get together for a neighborhood party, build in an activity. That can be as easy as a scavenger hunt, going ice skating, or a "field day" with fifty-yard dashes and relay races. Have parents and children alike join in. Keep it simple; just get people moving.

- **Create neighborhood activity nights.** Coordinate a weekly or monthly event, like a game of kickball, softball, soccer . . . it doesn't matter.

- **Invite neighborhood moms for walking playdates.** Instead of a playdate where the moms watch the kids play, do something active. Push the kids in the stroller to a park or around the neighborhood. On a rainy day, consider doing a fitness video together while the kids play.

Hack 45
Temptation Bundle

Brussels sprouts are all the rage on menus today. But, let's be honest—they're really just a vector for butter. By adding butter . . . and bacon, we've made these mini cabbages the plat du jour that we all love.

Exercising may feel a lot like eating plain Brussels sprouts—but what if we found the equivalent of butter and bacon for exercise? Suddenly, instead of pushing exercise to the side, you'd be seeking it out.

Sounds crazy? It's not—and it's called temptation bundling (TB). In TB, you pair something you don't always feel like doing (like exercising), with an indulgence (like watching *Game of Thrones*).

In a Wharton study on temptation bundling, participants were assigned to one of two groups: (A) the TB group, who were allowed to listen to an addictive audio book *only* when they exercised and (B) the control group, who could listen whenever they wanted. Those in the TB group worked out at the gym 51 percent more! Follow the steps below for your own temptation bundles. (Oh, it sounds so naughty, doesn't it?)

- **Choose your indulgence.** What do you enjoy? Is it watching *Real Housewives*? A good junk magazine? Or a new music playlist? Choose an indulgence that you regularly look forward to.

- **Pair the indulgence with an exercise.** Choose an exercise that allows you to simultaneously do that indulgence. Listen to an addictive audiobook or watch *Game of Thrones* while you're on the treadmill, read your favorite junk magazine while you're on the stair-climber, or make a playlist of your favorite songs for running.

- *Only* let yourself engage in the indulgence while exercising. This is key. Whatever you choose, *do not* let yourself indulge when you're not exercising, or this falls apart. When my *People* magazine arrives or I hear a favorite running song (two of my indulgences), it actually makes me look forward to exercising. You'll find that happens for you quickly if you adhere to this rule.

- Update the bundle when its effect starts to wear off. This effect can wear off over time, particularly when your book ends, the show's season is over, or the playlist music becomes stale. So, refresh your indulgences as needed.

Finding the Motivation and Building the Habit

Hack 46
Build an Exercise Habit

We make more than 30,000 decisions every day. That's a lot, and research shows that it exhausts our brains. In fact, a study of judges showed that the more decisions they had to make, the more likely they were to choose the easier or routine decision.[1]

If you have to decide where, how, or *whether* to exercise every day, your most likely choice is to just skip it. Especially when you're tired or overwhelmed, it's the easier choice.

But your brain has a solution for this mental fatigue: habits. Habits are automatic little shortcuts, and they're key to incorporating exercise.

106

How to Use Habits to Make Exercise Happen

What is a habit? We use this word all the time, but do we know what it means? A habit is like a little computer program in our brain: a subconscious process that doesn't require a decision, mental energy, or willpower. In fact, 45 percent of the actions we take every day are not conscious decisions but actually habits.[2] In a habit, trigger (A) leads you to automatically respond with action (B): when you get in the car (A), you put on your seat belt (B), or when you enter your house (A), you take off your shoes (B). You don't have to convince yourself to take off your shoes; you don't even think about it.

What happens in the brain when you make a decision or create a habit? When you make a decision, the region of the brain called the prefrontal cortex (PFC) is activated. Remember what I've said before about the PFC—it's a more recently developed part of the brain, gets easily overridden by the primitive portions of the brain, and gets worn out by decisions! However, when something becomes a habit, the PFC doesn't have to control it anymore. Just like once you learned to ride a bike, you don't have to *think* about how to stay upright on the bicycle, you just *do*.

Why do habits matter for health changes? Leveraging habits is one of the surest ways to make healthy changes last. In fact, research shows that people who make more healthy decisions actually rely less on self-control, and more on creating good habits that don't require self-control at all.[3]

How do you create a habit? Creating a new habit requires three things: (A) a trigger, (B) the actual activity, and (C) a reward. Your brain is able to form new connections (a phenomenon called neuroplasticity), and when you're creating a habit, you're literally laying down new neural networks. That's why it requires effort at first—and some willpower—on your part to make sure that A is always followed by B while your brain creates the connections. But once that link is established, it will *become as automatic as riding a bike*, willpower not required.

- **Step 1: Choose event A (the trigger).** This should be something you already do or that happens regardless of choices you make.[4]

- **Step 2: Pair the trigger with a small exercise to start.** Stanford University behavior scientist B. J. Fogg has coined the term "tiny habits."[5] Because when you're first creating that habit, what matters most is that A is *always* followed by B. By keeping B small, you make sure it's something you can always do. You can always increase the amount of time you exercise later, once the habit is set, and it won't require nearly as much effort.[6] Think of building your habit like training a dolphin to jump: They don't start by jumping twenty feet into the air on day 1, but with tiny steps. They first learn to touch the trainer's hand, then to follow a pole, and then to make small jumps to it. Only after long periods of building these habits and small steps are the dolphins ever asked to jump high.

- **Always do the habit, even if you have to make the tiny habit tinier that day.** On the days you can't do a full step B, shortening it is better than skipping it entirely. I don't care if it's for three minutes—still *do* it. You want to maintain that step A → step B habit, and just doing it for a few minutes can keep a placeholder so that the link is not broken.

Trigger/Event (A)	Exercise (B)
TIME In the morning when you wake up, or at 6 P.M.	Run for 20 (or 10!) minutes Do five pushups
SETTING At the start of soccer practice While on a conference call in your office After putting baby down for a nap	Walk around the field for 30 minutes March in place (put your phone on mute) Do a workout video
ACTION/EVENT Upon arriving to the office After putting the kids to bed After loading the dishwasher After going to the bathroom at work After walking in the front door After school drop-off	Do a fitness class after school drop-off Take the stairs Go for a 5-minute walk Do a 7-minute exercise DVD Stretch before bed for 5 minutes

Hack 47
Reward Good Behavior

Think of training your dog to sit. During training, *every* single time he does something correct, he gets a reward immediately, such as a "good boy," a scratch behind the ears, or a belly rub. Just like your pooch, your own habits will be reinforced more quickly by always pairing them with a reward.

- **Log it.** You know how great it feels to check off something on your to-do list, right? Do the same with exercise. Every time you exercise, log it. The more progress you make, the more sense of accomplishment and bigger endorphin rush you'll feel. Studies have shown that people who track their success develop more confidence that they can succeed (scientists call this "self-efficacy"), which leads them to exercise more.

- **Congratulate yourself.** The human brain likes its equivalent of a belly rub. After you've exercised, mentally congratulate yourself, and let yourself savor that "win" all day long.

- **Use external rewards.** While you're waiting for the habit to really set, it's okay to use external rewards. For every seven days that you do the habit, consider getting a new pair of socks, water bottle, headphones, or other gear.

- **Visualize the process, not the goal.** You've likely heard of people saying they "visualized their success." But instead of visualizing your goal,[7] visualizing the process to get there may be more effective.[8] Envision yourself doing your A → B → C program to reinforce your plans and help you predict (and proactively address) any obstacles.

Hack 48
Make a Routine, and Put It on the Calendar

If you don't put exercise on your calendar, it will not happen. So, once you've chosen your trigger and exercise, put it in the calendar and keep it consistent. The more consistent your routine can be in always having A → B, the more quickly the habit will set. The key is to keep the routine the same, either daily or at a minimum weekly, so it's never a question of "When will I work out today?"

The moment that you have to decide "should I exercise now"? is the moment that it falls by the wayside, so schedule it in.

OPTION A: Daily routine	Work out at the exact same time every day (if your schedule allows, this is the very best for adherence).
OPTION B: Weekly routine	If your schedule differs by days of the week (like mine), create a plan that may differ daily, but is the same every week. **My routine (dictated by my carpool responsibilities):** Monday 5:30 A.M.: Run 3 miles Tuesday 5:30 A.M.: 7-minute HIIT* Wednesday 5:30 A.M.: Run 3 miles Thursday 5:30 A.M.: 7-minute HIIT Friday 5:30 A.M.: Run 3 miles Saturday: Run or hike with the family (on weekends I don't schedule in the time, to allow us to be a bit more spontaneous) Sunday: Run or hike with the family **Another weekly option:** Monday 5:30 P.M.: 30 minutes cardio Tuesday morning: Strength training (with body weight, at home) Wednesday morning: Rest/yoga and sun salutations Thursday morning: 30 minutes cardio Friday afternoon: Spinning class Saturday: Hike with the family or other fun activity Sunday: Rest ——— *HIIT (High-intensity interval training)

Hack 49
Lock in a Goal

We care most about our "present self" today; we don't have nearly as much empathy for our "future self." That's why it's easy to say, "I'll run every day next week" or "I'll start eating healthy . . . *tomorrow*." But our future self eventually becomes our present self, and next week's run or diet starts *today*, at which point, we try to worm out of it.

But you can combat that with "commitment devices," which are little genius tools that lock in our strong intentions and increase our chances of success by 40 percent.[9] Then, once the *future* is *today*, there's no weaseling out!

You may already do this in other areas of your life: if you set your paycheck to automatically transfer some portion into savings before you even see it, or have the waiter package up half your dessert before it comes to the table, those are commitment devices.

- **Sign up for an activity where your workout partner cannot exercise if you don't show up.** Agreeing to meet a friend to work out is a commitment device because she'll work out alone if you're a no-show. But to really up the impact, make it so you *have* to be there, or she can't participate. Think activities such as a tennis match, kickball team, team rowing, or another team sport. Or if you walk together, keep each other's shoes, so that you both have to show up.

- **Publicize your goals.** There's nothing like sharing your goals with your family, friends, or on social media to create some pressure to reach them. Not only that, you'll also get some encouragement to help you reach your goal.

- **Create a financial penalty.** Set a penalty yourself, or sign up for an app where you have to forgo funds if you don't exercise, such as Beeminder. The app stickK takes it one step further (it's evil but genius): if you don't meet the goal it will take your forgone funds and donate them to a cause that you dislike to create even greater motivation.

- **Schedule a session with a trainer or pay ahead of time for a class.** Both of these increase commitment and up the chances you'll make it.

- **Make it impossible to *not* go to the gym.** Need a specific pair of shoes or other equipment for work? If you can, store it at the gym periodically, forcing yourself to go to the gym in the morning before heading into the office.

- **Find your own.** Find others that work for you! Make sure that it's something that you cannot reverse or weasel out of last minute.

Hack 50
Make Exercise Convenient

Behavior scientist B. J. Fogg teaches that "only three things will change behavior in the long term. (A) Have an epiphany, (B) Change your environment (what surrounds you), (C) Take baby steps."[10] We've discussed baby steps, so now it's time to take on our environment to make exercise the convenient choice.

Your environment can either sabotage your exercise goals— or help them. Need proof? Blue Zones Projects founder Dan Buettner has shown how adjusting your environment makes healthy choices easier and even subconscious. Working with the community of Albert Lea, Minnesota, Buettner and the city built more walking paths, made parks more inviting, and systematized "walking school buses." They advised grocery stores to move unhealthy foods to higher shelves and to put healthier alternatives at eye level and within easier reach. By making these changes alone—*and never telling people to eat better or exercise more*—biking and walking increased by 38 percent. The population lost 10 percent of its body weight, and added an average of 2.9 years to their lives.[11] Health-care costs dropped 28 percent. As Dan told me on my radio show, you simply have to "make the active choice the unavoidable choice."[12]

- **Keep your exercise equipment ready and within reach.** Do you have to haul your bicycle from the basement every time you want to use it, dig for your tennis racket or inline skates, or find that your headphones are always dead? These little obstacles are enough to derail you, particularly if time is short. Instead, keep equipment ready and easily accessible. Store battery-powered devices where they charge, so that they're always ready (because getting ready to exercise and realizing your headphones are dead sucks).

- **Keep your workout space clear.** A pile of clothes on your treadmill will motivate you to do laundry, not to exercise. So, if you work out at home, make your workout space a sacred and clear space.

- **Make little changes.** Make shifts to your home that encourage even small amounts of activity. Get up to change the TV instead of using the remote, get out of your car to open the garage. Instead of yelling upstairs for a family member, walk up and talk to them. (I *know*. Revolutionary.)

- **Get a standing desk.** If your office will spring for it, have them get a standing desk for you, or one that you and other coworkers can share. Otherwise, buy an adjustable riser that lets you convert a regular desk into a standing desk.

- **Help your own community.** Expand your efforts to your neighborhood to campaign for infrastructure changes like those made in Albert Lea. Every citizen can do this—never underestimate your grassroots power! In my own neighborhood, the lack of sidewalk along a segment of a busy street meant that we couldn't walk to a local park. By pushing city officials, my neighbors were able to get not just a sidewalk but a separate crosswalk as well.

Hack 51
Kick-Start a Morning Exercise Habit

Sure, getting out of bed earlier can be tough at first, but exercising before breakfast can burn up to 20 percent more fat[13]—and make it easier to keep the habit.[14] Bonus? When your workout is done before 8 A.M., you have *all* day long to pat yourself on the back.

- **Set the thermostat to start warming the house an hour before you get up.** Chilly temperatures keep us sleepy and inclined to stay in our cozy bed. Set your thermostat so that the house is warmer by wakeup time, making you ready to kick off those warm blankets.

- **Set your alarm to play kick-ass music.** When I was studying for my medical boards, I'd psych myself up for a pre-study morning run by setting my alarm to play U2's "Where the Streets Have No Name." I'd wake up to a great memory of attending the concert with my BFF, which immediately made me feel more energized.

- **Keep your gym clothes ready.** If you have to spend ten minutes every day to find gym clothes, that's ten minutes to find an excuse to avoid it. Best-selling author and financial advisor Ramit Sethi kept skipping his morning workouts until he started setting his gym clothes on the floor by his bed, where he couldn't get up without stepping over them. He says that this simple change increased his gym attendance by 300 percent.[15]

- **Really just don't want to get out of bed?** Start a morning stretching habit. (Stretching is one of those places we tend to skimp but gets more and more important as we . . . *ahem* . . . get older.) Reach your arms up as tall as you can go, and your toes down to lengthen your body. Pull one knee at a time to your chest and hold for thirty seconds. Cross one knee over your opposite hip and hold in a twist stretch. Just getting your blood flowing can be enough to get you moving.

- **Guzzle water before your feet hit the floor.** As we sleep, we lose water through sweating and breathing, leaving us dehydrated. That makes you feel groggier and your workout harder. Drink about one liter of water when you first get up.

- **Turn on the lights.** Bright lights shut off your melatonin release and restart your body clock for the day. Look out a window at the sun (or go outside if you can), use an alarm clock that lights up (available online for around twenty bucks), turn your bathroom lights on bright, or just look at your bright smartphone screen.

When the Going Gets Hard

Hack 52
Create Contingency Plans

We did these for nutrition, and they work for exercise, too. In fact, contingency plans are more effective than motivational messages[1] when you're tempted to ditch your exercise plan. *Secrets from the Eating Lab* author and researcher Dr. Traci Mann says that people who have "if-then" contingency plans are more than two times likelier to stick with their exercise program.[2]

- **Step 1.** Identify what obstacles trigger you to skip a workout.

- **Step 2.** Proactively choose a solution for the obstacle. Remember, it's okay if your solution is shorter/less intense than your original plan. As long as your contingency plan still has you doing *some* activity, that's a win.

STEP 1: Obstacles That Lead to You Skipping a Workout	STEP 2: Solution (choose only *one*, so you can commit to it)
If I feel too tired to work out	Turn on my favorite workout music to get me going Lower the intensity that day Exercise for just 8 minutes Experiment with working out at different times of the day
If I run out of time	Put workouts on the calendar, to protect their time Do a shorter, high-intensity workout instead Walk/take the stairs whenever possible today or tomorrow to compensate
If I don't have childcare (or the babysitter falls through)	Workout with your child, push him in the stroller on a walk, put him in the bouncer while you do a video, or use him as baby weights (see hack #34)
If I'm traveling	Walk up and down hotel stairs, pack a jump rope, or do a 7-minute high intensity workout in your hotel room. Ask the hotel for a map of walk/run routes Pack a magazine or iPad with a show you love, and enjoy it while you're on the hotel gym cardio machine
If I accidentally leave my gym clothes at home	Keep a spare set at the office Go home and do a workout video, high intensity workout, or neighborhood walk instead

(Continues)

(Continued)

STEP 1: Obstacles That Lead to You Skipping a Workout	STEP 2: Solution (choose only *one*, so you can commit to it)
If I have too much work to do	Take 7-minute mental breaks and walk the stairs/go for a walk Read a work document while on a cardio machine Take a call with a colleague while walking

What Are Yours?
(use this space to identify your own obstacles and solutions)

Hack 53
Get on Track After a Setback

You had a goal, a plan, and the tools, but you still missed three workouts in a row. Or you caved to the cookies . . . the entire box. Now you're in "aw screw it" mode, which is a soul-sucking (and goal-destroying) place. In one study of people trying to lose weight, researchers told half of the group that the meal they just ate had blown their calorie limit (even though they really hadn't). That group essentially gave up—and ate 50 percent more cookies afterward.[3] Point? It wasn't the initial setback so much as their attitude of throwing in the towel that truly sabotaged their diet.

Whether the goal is diet or exercise, a single slipup can feel like a full-on defeat. But these self-sabotaging responses are far more damaging than the initial slipup. Get back in the saddle a.s.a.p.

- **Don't blame yourself.** Let it go. *Let it goooooo.* . . . It may be counterintuitive, but studies show that people who forgive themselves for a mistake instead of fixating on it are less likely to repeat the error next time.[4] Acknowledge responsibility—but ditch the all-or-nothing attitude. So, you missed a workout or two . . . or a few. You did not just sentence yourself to a lifetime of being unhealthy.

- **Remember your "why."** Remind yourself why you exercise in the first place. What does exercise bring you that you'll miss out on otherwise? Is it better sleep? More energy? Being a good role model for your children?

- **Restart as soon as possible.** Forget the idea of, "well, I'll restart the diet/workout plan tomorrow." No. You restart *today. Right now.* Although the first step back on track is always the hardest, each successive session will be easier, and you'll quickly feel the boost in energy, well-being, and sleep.

- **Look for the root cause of the slip.** Did you slip up because you set an unrealistic goal or tried to squeeze in too much? If you're continually missing your goal, don't interpret it as a sign of weakness; you may simply need to modify a habit or play with the schedule. The key is to not give up or blame yourself but to keep manipulating these tools until you find what works.

- **Do a back-on-track kick start.** Identify small ways that you can symbolically get back on track, right now:
  - Do ten pushups before bed
  - Go for a ten-minute walk
  - Jump-rope for four minutes after you put the kids to bed
  - Commit to eating cleanly tonight
  - Drink twenty-four extra ounces of water

Hack 54
If You Still Can't Muster the Energy

If your exercise routine is consistently derailed because you don't have the energy, you could be locked into a vicious cycle of inactivity, erratic body cycles, and low energy. Exercise actually increases your energy, but if you're too sapped to even start, you may need to look at other aspects of your lifestyle.

All these factors influence each other. Improve one, and you'll naturally improve the others.

- **Nutrition.** You don't have to do a full nutrition overhaul, but what are you eating during the day? Sweets and processed carbs will give you a quick rush but leave you drained an hour later. Replace them with whole foods, such as produce, nuts, lean meats, or good fats, and you'll naturally see a rise in energy—perhaps just enough to get you out the door to start exercising.

- **Grab a cup of coffee pre-exercise.** If you drink caffeine around thirty to sixty minutes before you exercise, you'll get the optimal effect, which includes less discomfort, pain, and fatigue. (Drink it with a glass of water to prevent dehydration, and make sure to take a pee break before you go exercise!)

- **Hydration.** If you're beat, the culprit may be dehydration. Aim to drink, in ounces, half of your weight in pounds. So, a 140-pound woman should drink 70 ounces of water daily, and an extra 4–8 ounces of water for every caffeinated drink.

- **Sleep.** If you're consistently getting less than seven hours of sleep, having the energy to work out can be extra hard. Aim for a simple, low-intensity exercise, and then review the Sleep chapter for hacks on solving your sleep problems.

- **Just start slowly.** If you're too tired for an intense workout, do something less intense, such as walking or yoga. Over time, your energy levels will increase from doing those less intense activities, and you can up your intensity as you wish.

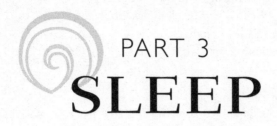

PART 3
SLEEP

Sleep Foundation: Structure

Sleep Foundation: Routines

Sleep Foundation: Environment and Lifestyle

Relaxation and Cognitive Techniques for Sleep

Troubleshooting

Child Specific Sleep Foundation and Troubleshooting

B efore we had children, we got a puppy, who we quickly realized had "digestive issues." By night I worked in the ER, by day I cleaned up after him. There was no sleep. Four days in, the vet offered to board the puppy while he completed his medications, and I said "Yes!" before she even finished. I called my mom as I headed home to get some rest.

Mom: You left your puppy at the vet?

Me: Yes. You can do that. Isn't it brilliant?

Mom: You know that when you have actual children, you can't do that, right?

(*Really? Like, is that a rule?*)

I'd love to tell you that "being a mom doesn't inherently make sleep harder," but I have an honest face, and you could tell I'm lying. In fact, well beyond the newborn stage, mom sleep takes a hit. In a study of women under age forty-five, *being a mother was the single determining factor affecting whether a woman was sleep-deprived.*[1] Add the fact that women are inherently more prone to insomnia than men, and there's a whole sisterhood awake at 2 A.M.

Because, if children were villains, sleep-sabotage would be their superpower. You see, sleep deprivation has long been used as a form of "enhanced interrogation" (a.k.a. torture), and I'm pretty convinced that children know this. I also read that the European Court of Human Rights called this practice "inhuman and degrading," *which made me question my newborn's ethics and sense of compassion when he was up at 2* A.M.

So, at least now you know *why* you start to go nuts when you're exhausted—it's a spy torture tactic. In residency we'd regularly have to stay awake for thirty hours at a time (it was *training,* not *torture,* I was told), and I realized that I'd never make it as a spy. I would have spilled nuclear secrets just to get a nap [CIA *agent reading this book* crosses my name off *spy list*]. Because sleep deprivation doesn't just play with our emotions and executive function, it disrupts our immune system and increases our risk of accidents, relationship discord, and weight gain. Children who have insufficient sleep are at higher risk of obesity, learning and developmental delays, behavioral outbursts, and even ADHD-like behavior.

On the flip side, as Amy Poehler tells us in her memoir *Yes, Please,* "One good night's sleep can help you realize that you shouldn't break up with someone, or you are being too hard on your friend, or you actually will win the race or the game or get the job. Sleep helps you win at life."[2]

The Two-Part Mom Sleep Two-Step

My mom was right: People look down upon asking to board your child at the veterinarian; sleep as a mom just isn't that simple. I can't just tell you to "prioritize sleep" and you'll suddenly get your ZZZs, as anyone who's stared at the ceiling at 1 A.M. can attest. That's especially true if your body's equilibrium or circadian rhythm are off.

As Poehler proceeded, "Sleep and I do not have a good relationship. . . . I am constantly chasing sleep and then pushing it away. A good night's sleep . . . is fraught with fear and disappointment. When it is just me alone with my restless body and mind, I feel like the whole world is asleep and gone."[3]

So to get your ZZZs, you have to address sleep from two angles:

1. **External** sleep saboteurs, such as your children and their sleep habits, your to-do list, late-night projects, and TV.

2. **Internal** factors, such as an out-of-sync circadian rhythm, stress, and racing thoughts.

The Internal Sleep Factors

Truth is, no matter how tired you are, you cannot *force* yourself to fall asleep. Harvard professor Dr. Daniel Wegner demonstrated a similar phenomenon in his famous "white bear" experiments. He told participants specifically *to not think of a white bear*.[4] Turned out, the harder participants tried to *not* think about the bear, the more they couldn't get it out of their head. Sleep is the same way—the more you try to force it, the harder it is.

Sounds impossible? It's not—with the right changes. Think of sleep like the hummingbirds my daughter likes to see on our patio. I cannot *force* hummingbirds to come, but, with the right environment, we can be pretty sure that "if you build it, they will come." So, I create an environment that is *hummingbird friendly*: safe, plenty of water and food, and they love to be there. We can't force sleep any easier than we can force hummingbirds, but if the environment is *sleep friendly*, then you'll finally get your own Field of Dreams—and the rest you need.

Sleep Foundation: Structure

What Is a Sleep Foundation?

A sleep foundation is just like the foundation of your home—get it right, and you're golden. Get it wrong, and you're facing leaks, varmints, and cracks in the floor. To build it, you'll need (1) a consistent schedule, (2) predictable routines, and (3) a pro-sleep environment and lifestyle.

Circadian Rhythm Jet Lag

If you've ever felt exhausted all day yet unable to fall asleep at night, you're "wired and tired." That feeling is common when your circadian rhythm is out of sync, or what's called Circadian Rhythm (CR) Jet Lag.

WHAT IS THE CIRCADIAN RHYTHM?

The circadian rhythm is your body's master clock, regulating the sleep/wake cycle, hunger, metabolism, and fat storage. Its impact on the timing of melatonin, cortisol, and a slew of other hormones

(Continues)

WHAT IS THE CIRCADIAN RHYTHM? (*Continued*)

is crucial for us to function optimally: melatonin needs to be released in the evening and overnight, growth hormone peaks while we sleep, and cortisol jumps in the morning and during the day. But if the CR is off, it's signaling these hormones to act at all the wrong times.

Living in CR jet lag is like trying to keep your schedule on Eastern Standard Time while you're living in Paris. An out-of-sync CR makes optimal health and weight loss practically impossible[1] and has been linked with mental health problems, gut issues, and even certain types of cancer.[2]

How badly does CR jet lag affect us? To find out, Harvard researchers studied the impact of waking up study participants at all hours to throw off their CR. After only ten days, their cortisol rhythms were completely backward, their blood pressure climbed, they slept poorly, and they had lower levels of the "fullness hormone" leptin, making them always hungry. *In fact, their health plummeted so much that by the end of the ten days, 30 percent of participants met criteria for prediabetes.*[3]

HOW DID MINE GET "OFF"?

Our CR adapted over thousands of years to sync with our environment, so that our ancestors could be awake during the day and sleep at night. That worked for anyone living before the 1900s, who rose and went to bed with the sun. But enter electricity and Netflix and *the interwebs*, and all that changed. Bright lights, late-night TV, and 24/7 devices mean that we're flooded with light long after the sun has set. Add in our erratic schedules (late to bed tonight, early tomorrow), and our CR has no daily stability or predictable schedule to follow.

WHAT DO I DO?

We've got you covered. We'll reset your CR by manipulating those same factors that threw it off in the first place. ZZZs are on the way!

Hack 55
Find the Right Wake-Up Time and Keep It

Your brain and circadian rhythm love a routine, so the first component of your sleep foundation is a consistent schedule. If that's predictable, your CR knows when to release (and stop) melatonin, making it easier for you to wake up—and to fall asleep more easily that night.

- **Set a regular weekday wake-up time.** Choose a single time and keep it consistent every weekday.

- **Aim for a loosely similar weekend wake-up time.** The closer your weekend wakeup time is to your weekday one (ideally no more than thirty to sixty minutes apart), the sooner your CR will sync. (Of course, if your small children are anything like mine, I'll see you Saturday morning at 5:30 A.M. sharp, regardless. Yay.)

- **The minute you wake up, get some light.** Whether it's sunlight outside or bright lights indoors, let bright light hit your eyes as soon as you wake up for your daily CR reboot (see hacks #58 and #62).

- **Stop snoozing.** If you normally hit snooze, set your alarm clock for the time that you *actually* get out of bed, and then do it. (No more snoozing. Sorry.) To move your wake-up time earlier, wait a few days until your body is accustomed to getting out of bed without snooze. Then slowly move your wake-up time earlier by ten- to fifteen-minute intervals every five days until you've hit your goal time.

- **Caveat for parents with many awakenings:** If you're sleep deprived because of your newborn or a sick kiddo's frequent awakenings (and otherwise have no trouble falling

asleep yourself), then aim for a loosely regular sleep schedule, but, honestly, sleep when you can. Read hacks #79–83
to get kiddos sleeping. Try to avoid making late weekend
wake-ups a pattern, since that can throw off your weekly
sleep cycle, but do what you need to do.

What Happens When I Sleep?

Sleep is divided into an average of five to six sleep cycles a night.
Each cycle lasts around 80–120 minutes and consists of NREM
and REM sleep.

NREM

- **Stage N1:** People unawakened in this lightest stage typically don't
  realize they were sleeping. (I also refer to this as "what happens
  to my husband when I discuss shopping.")

- **Stage N2:** Heart rate and breathing start to slow.

- **Stage N3 "Deep sleep" or "slow wave sleep":** N3 is our most
  physically restorative phase. Our muscles relax, our body se-
  cretes hormones for growth and repair, and we are out cold.

REM

- The majority of our dreaming occurs in REM, with active, awake-
  type brain activity. REM is our mentally restorative phase, where
  we consolidate memories and process events. Your body typically
  cannot move during REM.

What is a healthy amount of sleep? Seven to nine hours per night
is the sweet spot for most of us; some people need more, while
others (oh, you know who you are) need less.

> **How long should it take to fall asleep?** A normal time to fall asleep (called sleep latency), is around fifteen to twenty minutes. Less time means you're not getting enough sleep, while much longer means you're going to bed too early, have CR jet lag, or need to improve your sleep foundation.

Hack 56
Find the Right Bedtime and Keep It

My dad told me that when he was a kid his parents would occasionally let him stay up super-late to watch TV, and the TV stations stopped airing shows at midnight. So he went to bed because there wasn't anything else to do. Quaint, right?

For millennia, rising and sleeping with the sun kept our CR and sleep in sync with the environment. Not so today. For one, our bedtimes are later—there's just so much more to keep us awake! As Bella, a mom of three told me, nighttime is often her only adult time: "At times, I almost feel cheated of my adult time if I have to go to bed early. But then I'm woken up at 4 A.M. by my six-month-old, and I realize how much worse that would have felt if I had stayed up later." Later bedtimes are a main culprit behind why we sleep 20 percent less than we did a century ago, and why children sleep thirty minutes less than we did at their age.[4]

Our bedtimes are also erratic—late one night, earlier the next, and then super-late the following. Your CR can't even try to keep up and just goes haywire.

So, to set the right bedtime, it's important to pay attention to the *when,* and also to *consistency.*

- **Calculate the right bedtime:** Determine when you have to get up (say, 6:30 A.M.), then

  - *If you typically lie in bed at night for thirty minutes or longer,* set your bedtime for the time that you actually *fall asleep.* Get into bed about twenty minutes before that time. (See hack #59 for a bedtime routine to help you reset quickly and hack #75 for more on a later bedtime.)

  - *If you don't have difficulty falling asleep,* set your bedtime to allow for about seven and a half hours of sleep, and get into bed twenty to thirty minutes before that.

- **Keep it consistent—but the 80/20 rule is okay.** Just like your wake-up time, keep your bedtime within a thirty-minute window to allow for CR syncing, particularly in the first few weeks. The more regular your schedule, the sooner the CR can reset. After that, aim for the 80/20 rule: a late night here or there is okay when you're consistent 80 percent of the time.

Hack 57
Build Your Child's
Sleep Foundation Early On

Do not even whisper the words "baby" and "sleep" in a bookstore or around other moms. You'll be inundated with so many tips, advice, and promises that your head will spin, and you'll realize—like Ava Neyer did in her blog excerpted below, "I Read All the Baby Sleep Books"[5]—that there's absolutely no consensus.

Don't let your baby sleep too long, except when they've been napping too much, then you should wake them. Never wake a sleeping baby. Any baby problem can be solved by putting them to bed earlier, even if they are waking up too early. If your baby wakes up too early, put them to bed later or cut out a nap. Don't let them nap after 5 P.M. Sleep begets sleep, so try to get your child to sleep as much as possible. Put the baby to bed awake but drowsy. Don't wake the baby if it fell asleep while nursing.

You'd think that children haven't been sleeping for millions of years. You'd think that there's some magic unicorn trick that makes a baby a "good sleeper." Nah. It's time to simplify baby sleep.

Have you ever bought an appliance or electronic device—such as a TV—that came with both a Quick Start Guide and also the more detailed instruction manual (in five languages)? You open the quick guide—and it gets you going quickly. You can go to the detailed manual afterward if you need, but 80 percent of the time you get what you need with the quick guide.

That's the way baby sleep is. Jumping straight in with all the sleep philosophies and training practices and *miracle-sleep-fairy-nap-tips* is like jumping straight to the detailed manual *in German*—before you've even figured out how to plug in the TV. Put down the detailed manual. Let's start with sleep's equivalent of the Quick Start Guide, which is building your child's sleep foundation.

Once you've instituted a sleep foundation, many children will sleep well and not need any more guidance. For those who do, it's still much easier to troubleshoot or sleep train, once the sleep foundation is in place.

As LA-based certified child and family sleep consultant—and author of the upcoming *4 Pillars of Sleep Hygiene*—Jenni June told me, "Without a sleep foundation, none of the sleep-training methods will work. And even if it does, it will come undone when real-life circumstances come your way—such as travel and illness." Because the easiest way to minimize bedtime tears has nothing to do with "cry-it-out" or "no-cry" philosophies but everything to do with building a sleep foundation from day 1.

- **The sleep foundation components that work for you also work for your child.** Incorporate components of a sleep foundation as early as possible: a consistent schedule, stable wake-up and bedtime routines, a relaxing sleep environment, and plenty of physical activity and outdoor time. (We'll delve into each of these in detail shortly.) The exact components will change as a child grows, but the groundwork is the same.

- **Aim for a flexible routine, not a strict schedule.** Some baby books come with such strict schedules, you'd think they're for the Supreme Court, not a four-week-old. Every one loses their mind a little trying to adhere to these. Forget it. Instead, adopt a flexible routine where you still have a consistent general timing and order of activities but aren't fixated on the clock. Along those lines, once you have a good routine in place, the 80/20 rule is okay for the kiddos, too: if you're staying consistent 80–90 percent of the time, missing a nap or a late bedtime here or there is fine.

- **Limit their device time, especially two hours before bed.** As soon as your child uses a device, make a firm power-off time. Devices in the bedroom at night are linked with later bedtimes, less sleep, and poor sleep quality, so keep them out.

- **Thou shalt not listen to nonexpert "experts."** Do not—I repeat, *do not*—automatically internalize advice from your mother-in-law/neighbor/lady in the grocery line. They'll tell you how their child slept through the night at three weeks. *"I wonder why* YOURS *isn't doing that? Hmmmm."* Ignore that judgy vibe. *At three weeks postpartum, we're all such an exhausted, hormonal mess, we wouldn't know our baby from the Dalai Lama.* We don't remember baby's schedule twenty minutes ago; there's no way they accurately remember twenty years ago. Don't let them get into your head.

- **Good sleep takes a sleep foundation . . . and a little luck.** I say this because we moms internalize how well our children sleep (and eat, and poop, and burp, and . . .), as a critique of our mommy-ness. Keep doing your best, but know that some babies just sleep more easily than others. It doesn't make a baby a "good baby" or a "bad baby," or you a "bad mommy," it just . . . is. And, no matter what you do, it will change by next Thursday *because baby likes to keep you guessing.*

Sleep Foundation: Routines

Hack 58
Start a Morning Routine That Energizes

Earlier we discussed *when* you should wake up, now let's discuss what you'll actually do to get going. We all know that insufferable person who says she "wakes up at the same time every day, without an alarm clock." Don't hate her for her morning chipper-ness (well, maybe for a second); copy her.

- **Let in the light!** I know. I've said it before, but this single hack serves as your daily CR/body clock reset. If you're not getting a solid dose of light first thing in the morning, you're cheating yourself of the easiest way of waking up and resetting your body.

- **Hydrate.** We lose water during sleep and wake up with a water debt. Fix that immediately with 8–16 ounces of water. Make it more interesting with fruit slices, sparkling water, or herbal tea. I keep water on the bedside table, so it's in reach the moment I wake up.

- **Move! (even just a little).** If you're a morning workout person, bless you. If not, start easy. Go for a brisk walk or jog for ten minutes or try one of my favorite ways to start the day: sun salutations. My daughter and I do these to-gether, and she puts me to shame with her flexibility. See hack #51 for how to be a morning workout person.

- **Rock your favorite tunes.** Feeling like your get up and go got up and went? Get moving with tunes that build the music and have a strong positive beat.[1] Find your favorites, or search on line (many streaming services have wake-up playlists[2]).

The Power of Habit and Sleep

One year for my elementary school science fair, my mom helped me create a computer program: when you pressed the space bar (A), the computer automatically played the theme to *Star Wars* (B). (I know what you're thinking, and yes, I was obviously extremely cool.) We had created a simple A → B program, and your brain can do the same thing.

To manage everything that our brains have to process, the brain creates shortcuts by "chunking" activities together in A → B pairs. That means that when (A) (certain activities, thoughts, or emotions) occurs, your brain automatically reacts with an action (B)[3] without conscious effort.

Your brain will automatically create these programs if you re-peat the A → B pattern often enough (which is also how you form bad habits unintentionally). Or you can intentionally "program" your brain to create *good* habits (see hack #46 for more on habits).

When it comes to sleep, we'll initiate positive sleep habits and break the subconscious negative ones keeping you and your child awake. For each of these, we'll create an A → B program, where just starting the habit (A) triggers your brain to slow down and prepare for sleep.

Hack 59
Create Your Own Nighttime
Power-Down Routine

Your brain is not a car, and sleep isn't as simple as "hitting the brakes." In fact, it's more like letting your foot off the accelerator and the car eventually rolling to a stop. Which is why, if you're running 75 mph right up until you get into bed, you've got a while to coast before you can fall asleep.

A good bedtime routine gives you time to slow down, but it's more important than that; by creating a bedtime routine habit, you're writing an A → B program. Over time, just starting your bedtime routine (A) will cause your brain to automatically start to slow down (B). You'll more easily fall asleep and sleep more soundly. Try one like this routine from Dr. Michael Breus, author of *The Power of When*.

Just like with the kiddos, keep your routine to less than sixty minutes, or you'll lose the linkage between starting the routine and sleep.

- **Choose an event (A) to start the routine, one hour before bedtime.** Some people set their phone or watch alarms for a gentle ring when it's time to start the routine. Then put your phone away for the night. Mentally tell yourself, "Okay, now my bedtime routine starts" to establish it as the event (A).

- **Prep for the next day (ten minutes).** Gather lunches, set out clothes, pack bags, or finish up any last-minute needs.

- **Wash up (twenty minutes).** Wash your face, take a warm shower if you want, put on pj's, and get yourself otherwise ready for bed.

- **Relax (twenty to thirty minutes).** This is your time, so choose what relaxes you.

  - **Stretch, breathing, or yoga.** Do a few stretches while taking deep breaths (such as a standing forward bend, sitting with legs crossed and rolling your neck, or child's pose). (See hack #71 for more ways to relax your body.)

  - **Watch TV.** Yes, it's totally fine to watch TV if it relaxes you. Just avoid anything that you find really engaging/edge of your seat (e.g., *Gone Girl* may not be the best thing to watch before bed).

  - **Read something relaxing.** Just like TV, avoid stimulating reads, and opt for something calming. A good book, spiritual readings, or the Bible can all help you wind down. (Personally, nothing helps me sleep better than reading articles in my husband's sports magazines.)

  - **Gratitude.** Write down one or two things for which you are most grateful today.

  - **Play music, meditate, or whatever else relaxes you.** Anything that turns your brain off is good—bonus points if it feels even a little indulgent.

Hack 60
Create a Nighttime Routine for Your Child

A bedtime routine is about more than just getting kiddos washed and into pj's; young children are just learning how to fall asleep, and the bedtime routine is a cornerstone of their sleep foundation. A solid bedtime routine creates that A → B sleep program for them, too, helping them relax into sleep instead of fighting it.

Our one-year-old had suddenly started to struggle with sleep, and we realized that in the busyness of our evenings, we had started to short-change his bedtime routine (sorry, second child). We got back on track and were reminded of the power of sleep habits—for even our littlest ones.

Use the tips below for a general bedtime routine (see hacks #80–83 for specifics by age).

- **Choose the right bedtime.** Your child's bedtime depends on her own body timing, sleep needs, and your family's schedule. If mom or dad doesn't get home every night until 8 P.M., a 7 P.M. bedtime may leave everyone frustrated. On the contrary, evening meltdowns may signal needing an earlier bedtime. Pay attention to your child's signs of sleepiness, and choose a schedule that works for everyone.

- **Select a bedtime routine start time.** Once you've chosen bedtime, subtract fifteen to forty-five minutes (depending on your child's age) for the routine to start. Allow enough time so it's not hectic and rushed. For infants still feeding in the middle of the night, choose a late-evening feed after which baby naturally falls asleep as the "bedtime feeding," and build a small routine around that, so they can associate the routine with sleep.

- **Adjust as they grow.** For an infant, this routine is short (around fifteen minutes), while a toddler's can be thirty minutes (up to sixty minutes tops, including bath). Post a picture list of the routine so everyone can know what's next.

- **Keep it relaxing.** Once the routine starts, keep lights dim, and activities as relaxing as possible. Save the rambunctious hide-and-seek game for earlier in the day.

- **End on a favorite note.** Finish with the favorite part, such as story time or independent reading in bed for an older child. Having something to look forward to will help you progress through each of the steps.

Sleep Foundation:
Environment and Lifestyle

Hack 61
Don't Let Bedfellows Rob You of Sleep

Who sleeps in your bed? If it's a circus of you, your spouse, kids, and maybe a pet or two, it's not helping. Research shows that moms who co-sleep with children or pets experience more fragmented sleep and feel more tired and stressed. Of course, anyone awoken by a swift kidney kick from their three-year-old doesn't need research to know that. Reclaim your sleep-space.

- **For infants, share a room, not a bed.** According to the American Academy of Pediatrics (AAP), the safest place for babies under six months (and ideally, up to twelve months, per the AAP) is in your room—but not in your bed.[1] Put him on his back in a nearby bassinet so he'll be within arms' reach, but out of harm.

- **For older children, lovingly insist that they sleep in their bed.** Be firm that all sleep—including falling asleep and naps—happens in the child's bed. If you've gotten into a co-sleeping routine, experts suggest transitioning by sleeping on the floor of your child's room (which sounds like torture, so do yourself a favor and just don't start). If your child is sick and you want her close, consider putting her on an air mattress in your room instead of in your bed.

- **Keep bedtime conversations light.** Sometimes it feels like the only time we have to actually *talk* with our spouse is when we're getting into bed. Don't use that time to re-hash concerns or irritations. As my colleague Dr. Keith Roach says, "Anger murders sleep"; highly emotional topics before bed prevent falling asleep and reduce deep sleep. Save these discussions for long before bedtime.

- **Keep the pets out of bed.** I can tolerate only so many be-ings waking me up, so our dog lost all rights to our bedroom when baby came along. Have Fido sleep on the floor or out-side the bedroom altogether.

What External Factors Most Strongly Influence the Circadian Rhythm?

The downside to your CR being so sensitive to external factors is that they can easily disrupt it. The upside? You can deliberately leverage those same factors for a CR reset.

Of all the external factors that influence the CR (called zeitge-bers, you little science nerd), the most influential is light.[2] Light travels through the eye to the brain's suprachiasmatic nucleus,[3] which interprets bright light as a "WAKE-UP!" signal. It then shuts down melatonin release, raises body temperature, and releases cortisol—all to raise your energy and wakefulness.

That means that even if it's 11 P.M., if you're staring at your smartphone or are surrounded by bright light, your CR will sup-press melatonin release to keep that "awake" cycle going (mean-ing you'll have trouble falling asleep later).

On the flipside, that same bright light can actually help you in the morning. Looking at bright light when you first get up will send your CR a wake-up signal, start to energize you, and reset your CR for the day.

WHAT ELSE IMPACTS THE CR?

In addition to light, we'll later discuss how to leverage food, exercise, temperature, and even medications or supplements to affect your CR.

Hack 62
Optimize Daytime Light

Leverage light to help your sleep and energy by getting as much light as you can during the day. Then around three hours before bedtime, flip the script and deliberately minimize light, to prepare yourself for sleep.

- **Get bright light the moment you wake up.** Think of this as resetting your CR watch for the day. Go outside or look out the window if it's light when you wake up. If it's still dark (I hate you, daylight savings. So, so much.), look at indoor bright lights of at least 100 watts (such as bright bathroom lights), or even the blue light of your phone.[4] If you still have trouble, consider an alarm clock that lights up before your wake-up time, so the room becomes bright.

- **Get outdoor daily light.** Each hour of bright light exposure can shift the body clock by as much as thirty minutes,[5] so aim for twenty to thirty minutes of outdoor time every day (with sunscreen!). Aim for bright outdoor time earlier in the day if you have trouble waking up or later in the day if you're starting to get drowsy too early.

- **Consider a light box.** If you find that your sleep or moods are particularly affected by winter's waning light—consider thirty to forty-five minutes per day of 2,000–10,000 lux in a light box.

Hack 63
Cut the Evening Light

When I was a child, my family took a summer trip to Alaska, where the sun routinely set around midnight. My younger brothers and I thought this was *awesome!* We *never-wanted-to-go-to-sleep!!* My parents did *not* find that so awesome. We knew the clock said it was late, but we simply did not feel tired. Years later, I learned why: The late bright light was delaying our melatonin release.[6] *I also learned that I'm not taking my kids to Alaska until they're eighteen and can go to sleep (or not) on their own time.*

Children are even more vulnerable to bright light's effects on body clock and bedtime. In one recent study of preschoolers, researchers found that exposing them to bright light an hour before bedtime caused melatonin levels to plummet by almost 90 percent and to stay lower as much as an hour later.[7]

- **Turn down bright house lights during bedtime routines.** Keep ambient household lights (like hallways and other rooms) slightly lower during the bedtime routine and until after your child is asleep. Otherwise, bedtime stalling tricks like running out of their room will expose them to bright light, suppressing their melatonin release[8] and further delaying sleep. And *nobody* wants that.

- **Dim the bedroom bulbs.** In both kiddo's and your bedroom at bedtime, leave off overhead lights and only use bulbs that are under 40-watt equivalents (or around 400 lumens or 10 LED watts in the new bulbs) with no more than 300-watt equivalents total on in a room, advises Dr. Michael Breus. New LED bulbs emit even bluer light than traditional incandescent bulbs did,[9] so keep them off in the evening entirely. I designate a single small lamp with low-wattage bulbs in each bedroom, and that's all we turn on before bed (Breus recommends special bulbs with blue light filters called "good night" bulbs). Lights with a dimmer also work, as do fancy "smart bulbs" that change their hue to emit less blue light at night.

- **Use a book light.** If you or your partner reads in bed, use a book light instead of a large bedside lamp so that it doesn't bother the one trying to sleep. Also, if one of you uses a device, make sure it's dimmed.

- **Block even the little lights.** Even if a light isn't bright enough to consciously bother you, your brain can detect it through closed eyelids (see, moms *do* have eyes in the back of their heads).[10] With all the little blinking lights in our rooms (cable boxes, thermostat, alarm system, alarm clocks), it's like command central even at night. Turn them off if possible or simply cover them (I've used duct tape or an old T-shirt in a pinch).

- **Cover windows and doors.** If light is coming in through your windows, invest in blackout shades or darker fabric, and tack down the edges, too. If light comes around your door, apply a light-tight strip around its rim.

- **Mask it.** If light still bothers you, embrace your inner Holly Golightly and get a satin or silk eye mask.

- **Have to get up?** Avoid turning on lights if you can, but if you need a little light for a bathroom trip or to check on a munchkin, consider a nightlight with a bulb color designed for nighttime, or just a very low wattage (like 7.5 watts).

Hack 64
Harness Your Devices

As convenient as our smartphones are, they can wreak havoc on our sleep.[11] The blue light that they emit suppresses melatonin release even more than traditional white light and is a major culprit behind CR jet lag.[12] In 2013, the American Medical Association even issued a warning about the hazards of excessive bright light at night.[13] Kids are even more vulnerable: devices cause them to sleep less, have poorer-quality sleep, and experience more daytime sleepiness.[14]

Plus, what we read or watch on our devices tends to awaken us, whether it's a stressful work e-mail or the season finale of *The Handmaid's Tale*.

- **Set a smartphone curfew one to two hours pre-bedtime.** I will say it again: Put away all devices one to two hours before bedtime, for your children *and* you. For anyone having trouble falling asleep and getting up in the morning (called delayed sleep-wake phase disorder), this is even more crucial.[15]

- **Make bedrooms device-free.** Teens who text or e-mail after lights-out report substantially greater daytime sleepiness.[16] Create a charging dock for the entire family (say, in the kitchen or entryway).

- **Go analog.** Have something you need to remember or a pressing e-mail you need to send? Keep a paper and pen beside your bed to record these thoughts, so you can take care of them in the morning.

- **Just say no.** For heaven's sake, if you *do* wake up in the middle of the night or can't fall asleep, *don't* pick up your smartphone. You know you'll end up Facebook stalking someone, and that's never pretty at 2 A.M.

- **Rock some blue blockers.** If you must use a device at night, wear blue-blocker glasses and set your device to "nighttime" setting. Blue-blocker lenses block the blue-light wavelength, reducing its melatonin-suppressing effects.[17] They're so fly, they even have a 1990s rap song (go ahead, look it up).

Hack 65
Set the Right Temperature

Body temperature averages 98.6°F but follows a cycle: temperatures climb through the morning, dip temporarily in the early afternoon, peak between 7 and 9 P.M., and then fall again around 10 P.M.

That cycle influences our sleep, and when your body temperature falls, you start to feel sleepy (which is why you want to conk out during the afternoon dip).

Leverage temperature to help you sleep by taking steps to cool down in the evening and warm up in the morning.

- **Keep it cool.** A bedroom that's too warm keeps your temperature elevated, sabotaging sleep. Aim for 63°F–68°F. (If I just helped you win the thermostat wars, *you're welcome.*)

- **Lighten up pj's and linens.** If you wake up hot and sweaty at night (and not for *that* reason, *wink, wink*), your fabrics may be the culprit. Cotton is breathable but doesn't wick away moisture, leaving you sweaty. Consider moisture-wicking fabrics or even silk or new bamboo options, according to the National Sleep Foundation.[18] Save your money and stick to sheet thread counts of 200–400, as higher than 400 can trap heat.[19] According to Dr. Michael Breus, a comforter made of half-down and half-cotton will be juuuuust right.

- **Pillow talk.** Consider "cooling" pillows, which allow for more breathability.

- **Air it out.** A fan in your room will help with air circulation, keep you cool, and provide soothing white noise.

- **Take a warm shower before bed.** It may sound counterintuitive, but your body actually releases heat after a warm shower, cooling you and signaling your brain to prep for bedtime. Studies have shown that even a warm foot bath or hot water bottle at your feet can help (again, counterintuitive, but they cause you to *release* heat)[20] . . . *but does anyone younger than seventy-five actually use hot water bottles?*

Hack 66
Cut the Noise

How often have you been drifting to sleep when a noise or partner's snore jolted you awake? In fact, noise can disrupt your sleep even when you don't realize it: sleeping with someone who snores causes you to wake up more than twenty times an hour, although you're not even aware of the wake-up.[21]

- **Block the noise.** If your partner is willing to listen for the kids a few nights a week, put in earplugs and create a quiet sleep bubble. If the problem is your partner's snoring, get your lovable buzz saw to a sleep specialist; you'll both be grateful (see A Note on Obstructive Sleep Apnea).

- **Drown it out.** Consider a white noise machine or app; the same that you use for your child works for you. A fan can also provide white noise and a nice breeze.

- **Control the TV.** Partner watching TV at night? Invest in Bluetooth/wireless pillow speakers or headphones so you're not disturbed. If your partner falls asleep while watching

TV, setting the TV timer to turn off after a set time is more effective than the sharp elbow to the shoulder you may be *tempted* to do.

- **Silence others' alarms.** If your partner's alarm wakes you up before you need to, suggest switching it out for a vibrating alarm (they even have some that come in your pillowcase nowadays . . . I know . . . technology!) so that you're not jolted awake, too.

- **Consider relaxing music or sounds.** Relaxing music may help some people fall asleep more quickly.[22] Opt for spa-type music or sleep playlist options on many music apps. There's some evidence that binaural beats (sound waves played at different rates to your ears, available via apps) are as helpful as music. If you find the music distracting while you're in bed, consider listening to it while you're relaxing before bed and then shutting it off.

A Note on Obstructive Sleep Apnea

OSA is a condition that affects up to 30 percent of men and 15 percent of women, causing poor sleep quality, fatigue, and impaired daily functioning. OSA can also increase the risk of accidents and cardiovascular disease, so it's important that I mention it here.

Classic signs of OSA include snoring or moments of not breathing followed by snoring. Patients may also complain of waking up feeling like they're choking or gasping. Women may have more subtle symptoms, such as feeling like they're always tired even after sufficient hours of sleep.

If you think you or your partner may have OSA, speak with your physician to see whether you'd benefit from a sleep study.

Hack 67
Make Your Bedroom a Spa-Like Sanctuary

Is your bedroom a living to-do list: piles of clothes to be laundered, documents to be filed, and a dress to be hemmed? If so, it's time for an intervention. Think of the last time you visited a spa (yeah, it's been a while for me, too). Remember the muted colors, plush chairs, minimalist décor. . . . You felt more Zen and relaxed just by walking in.

With the right setup, you can make your bedroom a sanctuary. Over time, you'll create another A → B sleep habit where just walking into your bedroom will trigger your brain's sleep response.

- **Cut clutter.** Unless you live in a laundromat, you do not need piles of laundry in your bedroom. Same for piles of paper, items to be sorted, or anything else that creates a visual "to-do" the minute you walk into your sleep space.

- **Mute your color schemes.** If you have the time, channel your inner HGTV host, opting for soothing neutrals and unpatterned cool hues, avoiding bright colors or loud patterns. You can always let loose your wild, artsy decorative side in your living room, kitchen, or even your guest bedroom. (Guests can catch up on their sleep at their own house, right?)

- **Update mattress and pillows.** The National Sleep Foundation recommends changing your mattress every eight years and pillows every two.[23] Or use my unofficial rule of thumb: if you keep rolling down to the same divot in your mattress or if you wake up with a crick in your neck, it's time for replacements. When you go shopping, consider your specific sleep needs: memory-foam-type materials tend to hold heat,[24] while some mattresses and pillows may help you stay cooler. Also, consider your sleep position (back, side, stomach) when buying.

- **Use soothing scents.** Although your bedroom scents shouldn't hit you like a mall candle store, a little aromatherapy can help soothe the weary soul. Consider scents like lavender[25] or jasmine.

Hack 68
Minimize Food/Drink Sleep Killers

Food and sleep are closely intertwined: Studies show that your sleep impacts hormones that drive hunger, food cravings, and metabolism. But did you know that the reverse is also true—that what you eat also affects your sleep?

- **Avoid caffeine after 2 P.M.** That caffeine you had at lunch sticks around—as much as eight hours later. Avoid caffeine after 2 to 3 P.M. at the latest. If you're still having trouble sleeping, you could be a slow caffeine metabolizer, in which case cut it after noon. Our caffeine metabolism also slows with age, so be prepared to move that cutoff earlier as you get older. Remember that chocolate also contains caffeine (so sad).

- **Don't eat big meals within two to three hours of bedtime.** If you have a large meal just before bed (particularly if high in fat), your body will still be metabolizing it when you're trying to sleep, reducing REM sleep and increasing middle of the night awakenings.

- **Watch sugar, especially before bed.** Diets high in refined carbs and sugars are associated with poorer sleep,[26] but the culprit seems to be refined carbs, not *all* carbs.[27] So, if you want a bedtime snack, opt for complex carbs and skip the refined ones and candy.

- **Watch the alcohol.** Although alcohol shortens the time to fall asleep, it impairs deep, restorative sleep. Also, as the alcohol wears off, you're more likely to have sleep disruptions, nightmares, or sweating.

- **Avoid nicotine.** Much like caffeine, nicotine is a stimulant, making it more difficult to fall asleep and increasing nighttime awakenings. That includes not only cigarettes but nicotine replacement products as well.

- **Bedtime treats that *do* help.** Brew a little chamomile tea or opt for warm milk or an Ayurvedic blend of warm milk with a little turmeric, cinnamon, or honey thirty minutes before bed. The protein, carbs, and calcium enhance serotonin production and can help bring on slumber.

Hack 69
Exercise Strategically for Sleep and Energy

"And when the moon is on the rise, they all go up, to exercise!" Ah Sandra Boynton's *Going to Bed Book*—a bedtime routine staple. Although I don't advocate her before-bed intense exercise routine, regular exercise is mommy's little sleep helper. Aerobic exercise three times a week helps you fall asleep more quickly, have fewer middle-of-night wakeups, and more restorative sleep,[28] and quiet any bedtime racing thoughts.

When you exercise, your core body temperature rises and stays elevated; after four to five hours, it starts to fall—called the Thermogenic Effect. For the greatest sleep impact, time exercise to optimize that effect.

- **Try an afternoon workout to help you sleep.** When you exercise around 4–5 P.M., the Thermogenic Effect temperature drop will coincide with bedtime, triggering sleepiness. Of course, this time often coincides right with your child's afternoon activities, so consider a jog around soccer practice, ask to use the gym yourself during swim practice, or check out hack #38 for exercising with the kiddos.

- **A morning workout can help you get up in the morning . . . and sleep that night.** Exercising earlier in the day resets your body clock and gives you an immediate energy boost. Plus, research shows that women who exercise in the morning fall asleep more easily.

- **Avoid late-night physical activity.** Although exercise at any time of day will still improve your sleep, high-intensity exercise within four hours of sleep (well, except *that* kind of physical activity, but that's for another book . . .) can make it harder to fall asleep. If that's the only time you have to exercise, opt for activities such as walking, yoga, or Pilates.

- **Take a brisk walk outside when you're feeling sluggish.** This gives you the exercise-induced energy boost, plus the added effect of sunlight—a double whammy for energy. During my pregnancy, this was the only thing that kept me functional after 2 P.M. Take your favorite music or friend and power walk for five to fifteen minutes. You will be amazed at how much more alert you feel in the moment— and how much better you sleep that night.

- **Get your kids moving.** Researchers put activity monitors on 500 seven-year-olds (I get tired just thinking of analyzing *that* data) and found that the more children were active, the faster they fell asleep and the longer they slept. Aim for a minimum of sixty to ninety minutes of activity; don't worry about having to coordinate something organized; free play outside is perfect.

Relaxation and
Cognitive Techniques for Sleep

Hack 70
Harness Your Racing Mind

If your mind starts to race the moment your head hits the pillow, you're not alone. In fact, this is so common that some people start to link going to bed with anxiety, triggering what's called Sleep Dread.

Two things happen at night: (1) you have fewer distractions and more space to think . . . and dwell, plus (2) fatigue makes us lose perspective. So, you start to rehash the day's irritations, worries, and any other stresses—and everything seems like a much bigger deal at that hour. Before you know it, you're wide awake.

- **Designate a "Worry Time"/Worry Lockbox.** To get a hold on your worries, designate a five-minute window every day that you record them. Write down everything bothering you: financial concerns, fears about the future, or the snarky comeback you wish you'd thought of at the time. Then, when you're done, close it up, like locking up the worries. For one, when you see your concerns in black and white, you may realize they aren't as bad as you thought. Second, the next time you start to worry, tell yourself that you'll worry about it during your next worry time, but not now. If you just can't let it go, take out your journal, write it down, then lock away the worry again. After doing this consistently for one or two weeks, you'll find that these thoughts become less disruptive at bedtime.

- **Write down the *one* next step.** If you still find the thoughts worrying you, take the worry lockbox a step further by writing down *one* next step you can take for the issue that's bothering you. Converting a worrisome thought to an actionable step decreases its impact on your sleep.

- **Keep a notepad by the bedside.** Sometimes even positive thoughts can keep you awake. Just as we fall asleep, our mind can start to wander—sometimes coming up with creative ideas or solutions. So, keep a notepad at the bedside, so you can jot down any epiphanies and go to sleep in peace.

Hack 71
Practice Progressive Muscle Relaxation

During my residency training at Yale University, we would work shifts in the emergency psychiatry section, and one of the ER psychiatrists taught me this technique to help fall asleep. (Because if you want to see someone who knows a thing or two about stress, talk to an ER psychiatrist.)

Progressive muscle relaxation is based on tensing and relaxing muscle groups, and it has been shown to improve sleep quality and help people fall and stay asleep.[1]

1. **Get comfortable:** Sit or lie down.

2. **Tense the first group:** Starting at your feet, push your heels down, tensing the toes as you pull them up. Really feel the tension in your feet, shins, and calves.

3. **Relax the first group:** After five seconds, mentally say "relax" or "let go," and release the tension while you exhale. Notice the sensation of relaxation.

4. **Move up the body:** Now, point your toes. Feel the tension in the front of your calves for five seconds, then relax and exhale.

5. **Continue the tension/relaxation cycle while you move up your body:** Tense/relax the following groups: thighs/knees, stomach, upper back, arms and hands, neck/shoulders, and face.

6. **Repeat if necessary:** Repeat the cycle as needed, if you're not already drifting to sleep.

Hack 72
Challenge Your Thoughts

The more tired we are, the more we lose perspective. We start to catastrophize, causing even our smallest daily concerns to suddenly seem insurmountable. In these moments, your brain seems to reach for every possible worry, like some manic shopper who just won a spree at the grocery store and grabs everything that she can. Your tax bill? Definitely worth worrying about. That argument with your spouse? Yep. The snarky comment from your coworker? Throw that on the pile!

The problem with these inflated catastrophic thoughts is that we *believe* them at this hour and allow them to get us all worked up. But catastrophic thoughts are just thoughts—and not reality. It's time to bring back a little objectivity.

The solution? Cognitive restructuring, an effective component of cognitive behavioral therapy for insomnia (CBTi),[2] helps us regain perspective, challenge the catastrophic thoughts, and to replace them with truth.

- **In the moment say, "It's not even likely."** Our brains are amazing at coming up with worst-case scenarios. If you develop a new worry in the middle of the night, simply say to yourself, "It's not even likely." Just a small insertion of perspective can be enough to halt the train wreck of fast-brain thoughts.

- **Learn to challenge your thoughts.** Go through the table below and identify what concerns/catastrophic thoughts are your hot buttons. Then look at the data in the right column that challenges them. If none of the examples listed fit your concerns entirely, go through steps 1 and 2 yourself, and fill in the blank cells. Once you're done, keep this list handy to refer to it at night when these thoughts start to creep in.

- **Where to find more CBTi.** If you want more CBTi guidance, check out a sleep app with CBTi or therapists who offer it in individual or group therapy.[3]

STEP 1:	STEP 2:
Identify the root concern of the catastrophic thought. Ask yourself: What am I really worried about?	Challenge the Catastrophic Thought or False Belief with Truths, Facts, and Your Actual Experience. Is that belief or catastrophic thought even true? Is it possible that it's exaggerated or false? What are the chance that what I'm worried about will really happen? What has prior experience shown—when I worried about this in the past, what actually happened?
Example Catastrophic Thoughts:	**Examples to Challenge the Catastrophic Thoughts:**
If I don't get 8 hours, I cannot function at all.	**Prior experience:** "I actually feel fine when I get just 6 hours." **Facts:** Research shows that 7–9 hours/day is the sweet spot, and more than 9 may actually be worse than less than 7. We all need different amounts, so base yours on how you feel, not an arbitrary average.
If I don't sleep, I'll be exhausted and moody. I'll screw up the project, alienate my coworkers, and be fired. *Or* I'll be a crappy mom, my kids will hate me, my spouse will leave me, or I'll have a nervous breakdown.	**Experience:** "The last time I had a bad night, the next day certainly wasn't my best, but it was nowhere near as bad as I was dreading!" **Facts:** Although long-term sleep loss has negative consequences, tonight's alone will not. In fact, your negative *thoughts* about your sleep impact your mood more than the *actual* hours.[4]

Example Catastrophic Thoughts:	Examples to Challenge the Catastrophic Thoughts:
I haven't slept at all the entire time I've been in bed tonight.	**Fact:** Sleep studies show that people who have trouble sleeping habitually underestimate how much time they actually slept, thinking they didn't sleep a wink, when in fact they slept for several hours. (Particularly in NREM sleep, we are not conscious of being asleep, so we think we've been awake, when we've actually been asleep.)
I can't fall back asleep and I'm not going to get any sleep all night.	**Experience:** "Even on my worst nights I tend to get at least some sleep." **Fact:** Despite the effects of insomnia, the brain can somewhat adapt to sleep loss, functioning on 4–6 hours of what is called "core sleep."[5] **Fact:** It's not unusual to momentarily feel wide awake upon awakening, but you're likely to fall back asleep. In fact, as the night progresses, your chances of falling asleep increase further as your sleep drive accumulates.[6]
Write your own below:	

Hack 73
Do a Meditation for Sleep

I've never been one of those people who easily fall asleep; my husband is (and at times this makes me really annoyed). My sleep took a further nosedive when I became an ER doctor, working sporadic shifts with an overnight here, a day shift there—and no predictability to my sleep schedule. It became next to impossible to sleep when I needed. Just to get some rest, I started to reach for sleeping pills for a couple of weeks. But I knew it wasn't a long-term solution.

Until one night when I was traveling. I had switched time zones and knew sleep would be tougher, but I forgot the sleep medication at home. I started to get nervous, envisioning a sleepless night, when suddenly I remembered having read about mindfulness meditation for sleep. I was skeptical, but at this point I had nothing to lose. I got distracted several times during the meditation, but somewhere along the way I fell asleep and, the next thing I knew, it was morning.

Meditation evokes the "relaxation response," which helps people with insomnia fall asleep easier and sleep longer.[7] The effects of meditation are even comparable to the effects of prescription sleep medications.[8] As my experience shows, you don't have to be an experienced yogi to get the benefits of mindfulness meditation.

- **Follow a guided meditation.** For best results, I suggest following a guided meditation online or downloading an app (Headspace or Calm are two of many). See hack #102 for more on meditation.

- **DIY meditation for insomnia.** Lying in bed, focus on your breath. Breathe in through your nose, feeling your chest expand. Hold the breath, then breathe out through your mouth. Visualize the air traveling from your nose to your chest, and then back out. If you'd like, verbalize (mentally or out loud) "om," "relaxed," or another phrase with each inhale and exhale. If you sense your concerns starting to intrude, try to observe them, without becoming emotionally attached, and keep breathing through them.

- **If you're still not sleeping, value the time for relaxing.** Some studies suggest that instead of fighting your insomnia, simply accepting it can help your stress levels, if not your sleep. Arianna Huffington has said that when she can't sleep at night, instead of perseverating on the *lost* sleep, she thinks of it as *found* time to meditate. Take the pressure off falling back asleep by noting that even using the time to breathe gently and rest is beneficial.

Troubleshooting

Hack 74
Get Out of Bed When You Really
Can't Sleep

If you frequently find yourself wide awake in bed, frustrated and staring at the ceiling, your brain has built an A → B program— except that it's a habit that you don't want. In this instance, the trigger (A) is getting into bed, and the action (B) is to become anxious about sleep—which further keeps you awake. Break the habit by addressing A *and* B. First, use the relaxation techniques in the previous hacks to calm the stress response. However, if that doesn't work on a bad night, the next step is to break the pattern by removing yourself from the trigger (your bed).

Getting out of bed never seems like a *pleasant* option, but remember that you'd likely be lying awake, even if you did stay in bed. Plus, if you get up and only return to bed once you're relaxed and sleepy, you can break this connection over time, replacing it with one where you associate the bed with relaxation. And that makes it worth a try on your worst nights.

- **If you're tossing and turning, get out of bed.** If it's been thirty minutes or more, or you're simply getting to that mind-spinning, anxious place of not sleeping and feeling wired, get up.

- **Go to another relaxing space.** Go someplace comfortable and cozy that you enjoy. Keep the lights dim. Take a blanket; take some water if you want it.

- **Do a relaxing activity.** Wegner found that although telling people "don't think of the white bear" didn't work, giving them something else to focus on was effective. Read a book, knit, listen to music, use a favorite meditation app or one of the relaxation techniques from the previous hacks— anything that relaxes and distracts you. But, no matter what, choose something calming; don't watch *Homeland* or CNN; do not check Facebook or your e-mail.

- **Stay there until you start to feel sleepy.** Once you start to feel groggy and relaxed, go back to your bed and grab that shut-eye.

- **Repeat as necessary.** Even after you've broken the negative association, you may have future nights of similar struggles. When that happens, nip it in the bud by getting out of bed before it becomes a habit again.

Hack 75
If You Can't Fall Asleep, Start with a Later Bedtime

Many people who struggle to fall asleep try to compensate by getting into bed even earlier, which *seems* like a good idea. But trying to "game" your sleep that way is like getting to the airport for your flight four hours early: you won't take off any earlier, and all you're doing is waiting while your kids eat airport food and lick the waiting area chairs.

If you're still having trouble after implementing the get-out-of-bed hack, try this technique from insomnia therapy. You may get less sleep during this process because it leverages your fatigue to help you sleep, but it's only until you break the A → B link.

My friend Leah used to take two hours to fall asleep, so she'd try to compensate by going to bed earlier and earlier. By using this technique, she reset her sleep and now falls asleep around thirty minutes after getting into bed.

- **Step 1: Go to bed when you actually fall asleep.** If you go to bed at 10 P.M. but don't actually fall asleep until 12.30 A.M., then 12.00 A.M. is your bedtime tonight. At first, you will likely feel tired, but after several days (particularly if you follow the other hacks in this chapter), you'll find yourself falling asleep easily.

- **Step 2: Add back time.** Once you're falling asleep within twenty to thirty minutes, move your bedtime earlier by fifteen to thirty minutes. After five days if you're still falling asleep easily, you can move your bedtime earlier by another fifteen to thirty minutes. Go slowly, and if you start to lie awake again, push your bedtime later so that you don't resume bad habits.

- **No naps.** While you're adjusting your bedtime, avoid the temptation to take naps, which will just throw off your bedtime efforts.

- **Consider treatment for insomnia.** If you have persistent insomnia despite attempts to establish a sleep foundation or routines, I always advise considering further support. Cognitive behavioral therapy for insomnia has been shown to be very helpful, among other techniques you can learn from a sleep physician or specialist. Bottom line, support is available, and you don't have to deal with insomnia on your own.

Hack 76
Fall Back Asleep After a
Middle-of-the-Night Wakeup

I always had trouble falling asleep after baby's nighttime feedings—a challenge for many moms. No matter how soundly I was sleeping when baby woke, by the time he was asleep again, I was wired. As Dr. Michael Breus says, "The trick is trying not to turn on your brain." Next time you have to get up to feed a newborn, comfort a toddler, or simply wake up for no apparent reason, these tips will help you drift back to sleep.

- **Get up slowly!** For the longest time after my babies were born, when I heard them cry, I'd reflexively leap out of bed superhero-style, landing halfway across my bedroom, ready to break through walls to save my . . . oh wait . . . he'd fallen back asleep. I, however, could still feel the adrenaline flowing through my veins and would not be sleeping any time soon. If you must get up, do so slowly and try to keep your movements calm.

- **(If you can avoid it),** *don't* **get out of bed.** To fall asleep, your heart rate needs to be nice and slow. Standing up causes your heart rate and adrenaline levels to jump, waking you up, so avoid it if you can. If, for instance, you typically need something in the middle of the night (a glass of water, a cool cloth if you get hot, tissues to blow your nose), keep them at your bedside so you don't have to get up.

- **Put on slippers.** Who hasn't stepped on the cold tile in bare feet and felt that shock of cold? Keep warm fuzzy slippers by the bedside (and a robe if you need it) to keep you toasty and sleepy.

- **For heaven's sake, don't look at the clock!** Looking at the alarm clock in the middle of the night is like rubbernecking to see a bad accident: people know they won't like what they see, but they can't help but look. When we see the clock, we do mental math of how much sleep we're missing and start fixating on it, which wakes us up even more. Turn your alarm clock away from you or cover it when you go to bed, so you're not tempted to glimpse.

- **Don't turn on the light.** Use nightlights so you don't have to turn on bright overhead lights. Caveat: One night a friend of mine went to the bathroom but didn't turn on the lights and, in the dark, didn't see that her husband had fallen asleep sitting on the toilet. When she started to sit down . . . and felt hairy legs . . . she screamed enough to light up the state and started blindly swatting at her husband. Sleep fail. Takeaway? Don't fall asleep on the toilet. And if your spouse does, it may be safer if you ignore my no-lights rule. For your marriage's sake.

- **Stay detached.** Now is not the time to think about your to-do list, a frustrating conversation with a coworker, or any other thought rehashing. Repeat after me: "I will *not* pick up my smartphone." The combination of blue light plus the emotional engagement will erase any chance you had of sleep.

Hack 77
Use Sleep Aids Cautiously—or Not at All

Sleep can be so elusive. And it's tempting to just take a pill, which is why the number of twenty- to forty-four-year-olds taking sleep aids doubled from 2000 to 2004. Although sleep aids can be helpful for the short term, they build tolerance and dependence, which means that after regular use, you may have trouble falling asleep without them. Plus, it's not clear that they improve sleep quality: they may leave you less rested, at higher risk of accidents, and may even be linked to higher rates of death.[1]

New guidelines recommend making behavioral changes like the ones in this chapter first, as those changes alone for six weeks are as effective as taking a sleep medication,[2] and even better for long-term sleep.[3] If you still need help, use sleep aids for a short period at most, and then taper off quickly as the behavioral changes kick in.

- **Okay for the short term in specific instances:**

  - **Melatonin.** Science doesn't support melatonin as a long-term therapy, but if you're struggling with jet lag or a circadian rhythm that is shifted later (called Delayed Sleep-Wake Disorder), a short course of melatonin may help.[4] Take a small dose an hour and a half to two hours before bed. Because of potential impact of melatonin on growth hormone and development, speak with your doctor before taking melatonin if you're pregnant or nursing, or before giving it to a child.

  - **Prescription sleep medications.** If you're considering one of these medications, speak with your doctor about your particular sleep problem (trouble falling asleep versus trouble staying asleep, for instance), as different medications address these problems individually. These medications can lead to daytime drowsiness and cognitive impairment, so use with caution and only for a short time while you're also making other behavioral changes.

- **I'm not a fan:**

  - **Valerian.** Valerian acts on the sedation receptors of the brain, leading to a general drowsiness, but not necessarily any better sleep. Given the lack of efficacy and risk for added adverse effects,[5] I don't recommend it.

  - **Antihistamines.** These medications act directly on the histamine receptor, which has a side effect of overall sleepiness (in addition to several less desirable side effects). They also induce tolerance and residual drowsiness, which is why they're associated with increased risk of falling and accidents the next day.

- **Vitamins and minerals that may help sleep:**

  - **Magnesium.** Magnesium has potentially been shown to be helpful, particularly for women who have sleep problems associated with their menstrual cycle.

  - **Iron.** Iron deficiency has been associated with restless leg syndrome. Women who are menstruating or pregnant may be iron deficient, so if you're experiencing these symptoms, ask your doctor whether you should start on a supplement or have your levels checked.

  - **Calcium.** Calcium may have a relaxing effect on our nervous system. Take it in the form of a glass of warm dairy or soy milk before bed, which will also provide a nice dose of magnesium and potassium.

Hack 78
Nap Sparingly—and Strategically

Whether a nap helps or hurts you depends on the cause of your sleep deprivation. If you're exhausted because baby kept you up all night but you personally have no trouble falling asleep, go ahead and catch some shut-eye if you can.

However, if your problem is difficulty sleeping at night, then avoid naps since they can compound that problem.

- **A power nap.** If you're beat but have to get on with your day, opt for a twenty-five-minute power nap. Any longer creates sleep inertia (that groggy feeling) and reduces your sleep drive that night.

- **A sleep cycle nap.** If you have more time, you can use a nap to replace your sleep deficit. A nap of sixty to ninety minutes will allow you to get a full sleep cycle. The best time for a nap is usually around 1–2:30 P.M. (aim to be awake by 3 P.M.), to coincide with your natural dip in cortisol and rise in melatonin. If you've been up all night with a newborn, take what's called an "ultradian multiple," meaning long enough to include two sleep cycles, or around three hours. Thomas Edison, who long swore that he slept only four hours a night, also took one to two 3-hour naps a day. See? *Even he wasn't superhuman.*

- **A high-octane nap.** Dr. Michael Breus has what he calls the "nap-a-latte"—a power combo of a nap and caffeine for when you *really* need to power through. Brew a cup of drip coffee, adding a couple of ice cubes so that you can drink it quickly. Down the coffee, then take a twenty-five-minute nap. You'll wake up ready to take on the world. (He started doing this while he was studying for his boards and had a newborn, naturally.) Just don't do this after 2 P.M., or you'll be dancing on the ceiling (*oh what a feeeeeling*).

Child-Specific Sleep Foundation and Troubleshooting

Hack 79
Troubleshooting Baby's Sleep

Even with a good sleep foundation, most kiddos will need some help with sleep at one point or another (*I'm pretty sure that's because they don't want us to get overly confident in our parenting skills*). When that happens, it's time for a little troubleshooting.

- **Go back to your foundation (hack #57).** If baby isn't sleeping the first step is to double-check the foundation. Maybe the sleep routine or sleep habit slipped a little. It happens. Alternatively, a sleep regression may signal that the sleep routine needs to evolve as baby is developing new skills (see hacks #80–83 for age-appropriate changes).

- **Rule out an acute condition or discomfort.** If baby's struggling to rest, make sure that he isn't dealing with an uncomfortable medical condition like a cold, reflux, or teething (ask your pediatrician if you aren't certain). Babies need more soothing during those times, plus, unless you first treat the condition, no amount of crying will create a sleep habit. According to Dr. Tanya Altmann, pediatrician and author of *Baby and Toddler Basics*, "Many times when sleep nurses are called in to help sleep train a baby, they'll realize that something else is going on, like reflux. In those cases, the baby needs to have the condition treated. Once that's done, the sleep issues may improve themselves, and if not, you can try again once baby is better."

- **Try moving bedtime.**

  - **Put baby to bed earlier.** If baby is having tantrums at bedtime, she may be just overtired. Try to have the bedtime routine complete and baby in bed just before the time she typically tends to show "sleepy signs" (being quiet, calming, spacing out a little bit[1]) to head off meltdowns.

  - **If baby's not unhappy but just wide awake, flip the script and try a faded bedtime.** With faded bedtime, you leverage the time at which your child naturally seems sleepy to create a habit. Set that as a temporary bedtime (even though it may be later), and finish the routine right around that natural sleepy point. After a few days, your child will create the A → B link between the routine and sleep. Once that link is set, you can move bedtime ten to fifteen minutes earlier every few days until you reach the desired time.

- **Keep sleep-training methods consistent.** Don't do controlled crying one night, and then have baby sleep in your arms the next, or he won't understand why crying leads to attention some days but not others. (See A Word on "Sleep Training.") That doesn't mean you can't change, but just don't switch back and forth.

- **If you need help, speak to your pediatrician or a sleep specialist.** Sometimes you can do everything "right," but kiddo just isn't sleeping well. When that happens, talk to your pediatrician for further suggestions or to see whether a sleep specialist would be helpful.

A Word on "Sleep Training"

People can get really passionate about sleep-training methods, and when you're standing there with moms or in the bookstore, it can feel like you have to "choose a side." Ugh—suddenly, it feels like baby sleep is a battlefield (and here you thought that was just "love"). So, to new parents worrying about this, I have three points: (1) try not to stress too much about labels, (2) do what feels right, and (3) see below for more info.

There are dozens of sleep-training philosophies, and they essentially all fall along a continuum, based on how much parents are actively involved in soothing the child. (Note: I refer to all of them as "sleep training" even though that term is often used as a shorthand for Cry-It-Out, because they're all teaching baby to sleep.)

Getting into all the sleep philosophies is beyond the scope of this book, but if your kiddo is struggling to sleep after doing the above sleep foundations and habits, here's where to turn next.

1. Start with "No/Minimal cry" sleep-training methods. I recommend that most parents start sleep training here, as many will find the solutions that they need. Granted, these can take longer to work (and require more work, in general), but with fewer tears, which makes everyone happy. Examples include Dr. William Sears (*The Baby Book*) and Elizbeth Pantley (*The No-Cry Sleep Solution*). (Note: These are sometimes also referred to as "positive" or "gentle" methods.)

2. When to consider other methods. For some families, No/Minimal cry methods may not be enough to get everyone sleeping well. Or maybe they worked for a while, but now bedtime is a struggle. If that happens, particularly if a child is older and his poor sleep is potentially becoming disruptive, then methods that tolerate crying (often referred to as "Cry It Out") may be helpful. Examples include Dr. Richard Ferber (*Solve Your Child's Sleep Problems*) or Dr. Marc Weissbluth (*Healthy Sleep Habits, Happy Child*). (Note: you'll also hear phrases such as "controlled crying," "graduated extinction," and "rapid extinction" to describe these methods.) Be careful not to start these too early, however: before six months or so, babies don't understand cause and effect, nor do they have the sleep foundation for the process to hold. That means you'd likely have to redo Cry-It-Out again when he's older (and no one wants that).

Most of all, listen to your gut. We say in medicine, "no baby reads the books," meaning no baby exactly follows the textbook patterns. Don't drive yourself bananas over it. Don't agonize over trying to make baby "fit" some book's rigid sleep schedule, or to implement a method that doesn't feel comfortable. Worry less about the labels, and focus most on what feels best for you and baby.

And one quick note from your friendly ER doctor: While we're here, I wanted to mention, one of the most powerful signs I hear in the ER is a parent telling me "something isn't right." No one knows your child better than you, whether that's regarding sick symptoms, behavior, or sleep training.

If something doesn't feel right for you and your baby, then it isn't—don't ever question or apologize for your mommy sense.

Hack 80
Newborn to Six Weeks

Whoever coined the phrase "sleeping like a baby" clearly never had a newborn. Sleep in those first few weeks is chaotic at best: fourteen to eighteen hours total daily sleep divided into intervals ranging from thirty minutes to four hours. Also, a newborn's circadian rhythm isn't yet developed, so she has no qualms about waking you up at night, a fun phenomenon known as day-night reversal.

Newborn and Infant Sleep Architecture

The sleep structure of newborns and children differs significantly from an adult's; understanding those differences can help address their sleep challenges.

For one, newborn sleep cycles are short. Unlike yours, which are 90–120 minutes, newborn cycles last 50 minutes, and they spend more time in REM sleep, during which they're more active and sleeping lighter. Not only are they more easily awoken while they're sleeping, more frequent cycles mean more chances to wake up overall. An infant is especially easily awoken in the first 20 minutes of sleep, so wait 20–25 minutes if you need to move the baby (or until you see his body relax without any twitching).

Babies don't sleep this way to frustrate you (*promise*). It's because it's necessary for their survival. More frequent and easy arousals protect against sudden infant death syndrome (SIDS). When babies sleep deeply, they're less able to arouse themselves (and breathe deeply) if life-threatening problems such as low oxygen occur.[2] So, in the newborn stage where vital systems are still developing and a little unstable, frequent arousals are a *good* and protective thing.

As babies grow, their sleep architecture evolves, too. They fall into deep sleep faster, have more deep sleep overall, and sleep cycles lengthen. Meaning they'll soon start to sleep longer. And you will, too.

Without a CR to govern their sleep, newborns rely on their unique sleep architecture (see Newborn and Infant Sleep Architecture) and their basic physical needs: hunger, dirty diapers, or needing soothing, to govern when they sleep and wake.

So baby won't sleep according to your day planner, but that doesn't mean you're out of luck. Just like your own CR and sleep cycles are influenced by external cues that you can leverage to help you sleep, so are your newborn's.

- **Quick Point: You cannot spoil a newborn.** Human babies are born far more vulnerable and dependent on their parents than any other mammal. Giraffe babies walk shortly after birth. (*They also weigh 10 percent of their mother's weight at birth,*[3] *which would be like having a fifteen-pound baby, so just thank Mother Nature for that one.*) Many pediatricians and child experts refer to the first three months of baby's life as the "fourth trimester," during which baby needs a caregiver's presence more frequently. Don't worry about spoiling your newborn; she doesn't even understand cause and effect at this stage. Love on your baby as much as you can during this time, and when you need to relax her, use techniques that mimic the nurturing feeling of the womb (see Leverage Tried and True Baby-Soothing Techniques).

- **Aim for a consistent but flexible routine—*not* a strict schedule.** I've seen many a mom distraught that she's "failing" because she can't keep her newborn on the strictly

timed schedule she read about. Nonsense. Jenni June
notes that she gets calls from moms all the time to sleep
train their infants at this stage —but they're just unable to
do timed training this early. Your newborn baby does not
read time; his body simply isn't built for that right now.
Follow baby's natural body clock for on-demand feeding
and sleeping during this early time, and use flexible routines to start laying the groundwork.

- **From day 1, institute a difference between day and
  night.** Although baby's CR won't start to settle until around
  six to twelve weeks, you can help it along by creating small
  differences between day and night from day 1. Reserve the
  day for playtime, activities, tummy time, and plenty of sunlight. Keep daytime naps shorter than three hours, and
  make nighttime feedings dark (using only a closet light or a
  lamp), calm, and boring (no playtime/fun activities).

- **Start a small bedtime routine.** When baby is eating
  every two or three hours, no one time may seem like "bedtime." So, designate an evening feed (around 7 or 8 P.M.)
  after which she typically falls asleep as "bedtime." Do a
  mini-routine of a short bath, pj's and swaddle, breast or
  bottle, and bed to start creating the bedtime routine
  habit.

- **Choose the right sleep spot.** In the first six to twelve
  months, having baby sleep in your room—but not in your
  bed—cuts his risk of SIDS by 80 percent.[4] Emphasis on
  the not-in-your-bed part: having baby sleep in your bed
  quadruples his risk of SIDS,[5] so use a certified safe bassinet, crib, or co-sleeper. It's okay to bring the baby into
  bed with you for nursing, cuddling, and reading books,
  but when it's time to sleep, place baby in his own sleep
  space.

- **Arrange for support from day 1.** When you're planning your hospital go-bag, plan how you'll have support. You *are* a super mom. You are not superwoman. Whether that's a spouse, grandparent, friend, nanny, or night nurse once a week or more regularly, take any help that you can. On the nights you have help, your support person brings the baby to you to nurse but otherwise handles everything else (changing diapers, soothing back to sleep). Once your milk and baby's latch are established, or if you're feeding formula, that person can bottle-feed baby and let you sleep. Another option is to take shifts: you respond to the baby from 9 P.M. to 2 A.M., and your support person takes over from 2 A.M. to 7 A.M.

Tried and True
Baby-Soothing Techniques

TRY SKIN-TO-SKIN CONTACT

You've heard about the benefit of skin-to-skin contact right at delivery, but new research suggests that the benefits extend far beyond the first few days and affect not only mother-child bonding but also brain development. BTW, Mom's not the only one who can do this—partners and grandparents can do skin-to-skin, too!

THE 5 S'S

Dr. Harvey Karp, author of *Happiest Baby on the Block*, uses the 5 S's[6] to mimic the security baby felt in the womb. (See his popular baby-soothing videos for more details):

Swaddle	Shush
Side or stomach position	Swing
	Suck

(Continues)

(Continued)

Tried and True
Baby-Soothing Techniques (Continued)

OTHER RELAXING TECHNIQUES

Pacifiers, sound machines, baby massage, car rides, singing to your baby, and rocking him are all other techniques to help calm a fussy baby. If you need to get things done and baby won't let you put him down, put him in the baby carrier on your chest and proceed. Many a mom will find that being close to you was all baby needed. Every baby is different, and sometimes your baby will need a combination of several of these, so they're good to have in your mommy tool kit. Remember, in this "fourth trimester," anything that can replicate the safety and coziness of the womb may help.

Hack 81
Six Weeks to Five Months

The day you see baby's first real "social" smile (not just passing gas but a bona fide smile) is a milestone—and not just because your heart melts. Grab the bubbly because this smile means that baby's reached a development stage where both her circadian rhythm starts to develop[7] and her tummy grows a little bigger (even though she'll likely still need to eat overnight), so she can sleep for slightly longer stretches.

Fist-pump! Keep building on that sleep foundation because in this stage the habits can really start to take hold.

- **Give baby a stretch of active awake time before bedtime.** Aim for an active awake interval in the evening before his bedtime routine and (what you hope will be) a longer interval of sleep. Give him some tummy time, playtime with toys, lying in a bouncy seat or on a kick and play mat. Letting him play, kick, and reach for hanging toys burns a little energy and further establishes the night/day difference.

- **Look for sleepy signs.** If you put baby to sleep when she's overtired, she's more likely to struggle with sleep and need your help; get her to sleep at the right time, and sleep will be easier. Look for subtle sleepiness signs, such as yawning, being quiet or less interested in the things around her. If baby's doing those things, get her to bed ASAP, and then tomorrow have her bedtime routine finished just before the time these signs typically start.

- **Try putting him in the bed when sleepy but awake.** If baby is full, happy, and has eyes that are at half mast, try to lay him in the crib sleepy but awake. Getting him used to this pattern early on may make it easier for him to learn to fall asleep on his own. Some days this will work like a charm; others it won't. That's okay; babies don't behave the same way every day, so any time that you get him to successfully fall asleep on his own is a win.

- **Don't scoop him up the moment he stirs.** Babies often stir during their active sleep, but it doesn't mean they're awake. Resist the urge to run in immediately, in case she's just actively sleeping.[8] Plus, even if baby is awake, if she's calm and isn't crying, she may fall back asleep on her own. As Dr. William Sears told me, "When your baby wakes up, the first thing you should ask yourself is, "If I were my baby, how would I want my mother to react?" Go in if she seems upset or like she needs you, but if she's not, give her the chance to see whether she can transition back to sleep without you.

- **Surviving colic.** Colic refers to those moments (or some-times hours or days) of baby being fussy with no apparent reason. Colic tends to peak around six to eight weeks, and although most kids will have outgrown it by four to six months, it's a *really hard* period. If you have a fussy baby, talk with your pediatrician to rule out medical causes, as well as to see whether she can suggest resources (some pe-diatric practices even have "fussy baby clinics"). Try baby relaxation techniques (see Leverage Tried and True Baby-Soothing Techniques)—and you really need to hear this— make sure to give yourself a break. If you've reached a breaking point and you're alone, set him safely in the crib and take a five-minute breather. *He is perfectly safe in his crib. Call a loved one or other support. You are doing a great job, mama. Please remember that I said so.*

Hack 82
Five Months to Fifteen Months

Good news! You've rounded a corner: You're now beyond the "fourth trimester." (*Pats back. Does dance.*) By five months, ba-by's sleeping and eating patterns are more consistent, she's holding her head up and interacting more, and even learning cause and effect. By the time you reach fifteen months, you have a toddler! . . . um . . . *congratulations?*

During this phase, the CR will truly establish itself, plus baby will really be able to start longer periods of deep stage 3 sleep, meaning the start of a more predictable schedule and fewer nighttime arousals. New challenges will arise (because this is life) in terms of sleep regression and teething, but by six months, many infants are able to sleep five to seven hours at night! Some may sleep even more, *but if that's your child, just keep it to yourself, and don't rub it in, okay?*

- **Protect baby's sleep.** Previously, you were able to cart baby around with you everywhere. But now you want him to learn to sleep for multiple sleep cycles and into deeper stage 3 sleep without relying on you. That requires an environment conducive to sleep, particularly when transitioning from one sleep cycle to the next. So, try to be as protective of naptime as you can as she learns this skill.

- **Consolidate naps.** Transition from more frequent, shorter naps to two longer naps daily, ideally around 9 A.M. and 1 P.M. If at first baby has trouble staying awake that long, engage him in stimulating activities because the longer awake interval will facilitate the longer nap.

- **Cement a bedtime routine.** Further build on your bedtime routine: bath, pj's, milk and a bedtime story, cleaning gums or brushing teeth, then kisses/hugs/prayers, and bedtime. For baby to build that A → B link between the routine and sleep, keep routines less than thirty minutes (sixty minutes, tops, if it includes a bath time). Incorporate any habitual stalling techniques directly into the routine (such as potty, a drink of water, or checking under the bed) to keep them from delaying bedtime.

- **Deal with "sleep regression."** Jenni June told me that, in fact, this "is not a regression at all, it's a progression. But parents are still responding with things that worked for the first four months that don't work anymore." Baby is outgrowing the sleep skills she has developed and needs your help learning new ones. To help her learn to connect one sleep cycle to the next, make sure the temperature is appropriate, and that she's not being awoken by household noises. Also, limiting the morning nap to around fifty minutes can help.[9]

- **Keep up the activity.** Make sure that your kiddo is getting adequate time for physical activity. One driver of sleep regression occurs when your child is about to transition to crawling or walking but just isn't able to physically do it yet. So make sure that baby's getting plenty of activity and outdoor time, whatever his capability. Allow him to get exercise with the bouncer, play on the kick mat, crawl if he can, and other stimulating activities. My beloved childhood babysitter used to say we'd sleep better if we "got wore out" with activity. She was right.

- **Deal with teething.** Because growth hormones are released during sleep, babies often feel more teething discomfort at night. Signs of teething include drooling, increased biting/chewing, or even inflamed gums with teeth erupting. If your child seems particularly uncomfortable, ask your doctor about giving an appropriate dose of a pain reliever such as acetaminophen or ibuprofen (after six months).

Hack 83
Sixteen Months to Four Years

You're now firmly grounded in the toddler years. Baby will be walking, talking, and growing into a little human being! Sleep will continue to consolidate further, and most kiddos drop to one nap around twelve to fifteen months. In fact, 75 percent of children drop their naps altogether by age three and a half. (I know, *le sigh*.)

As your child makes these changes and transitions from crib to a bed, it's also a crucial time to cement that sleep foundation and troubleshoot negative sleep habits while she's still young.

- **Consider sleep conditioning/training if your child is still unable to sleep on his own.** A time and place for everything, right? If your child has a good sleep foundation but is still having trouble falling asleep or unable to sleep without you, have a conversation with your pediatrician to troubleshoot. It's okay if your child doesn't follow the sleep books, but if he's nearly two or two and a half, and has a sleep pattern that's difficult or disruptive, it may be time to consider a sleep-training process to establish good sleep patterns.

- **Alternate "nights off" with your partner.** Even though you may not have baby waking up to feed anymore, children still wake up at night (bathroom, water, nightmare), and many moms—myself included—suffer from sleep-disrupting hypervigilance. To turn that off, designate a few nights a week that your partner responds to the kiddos. On those nights, put in your earplugs, turn off your mommy vigilance, and get some rest.

- **Limit screen time.** Munchkins often start using devices during this time. The American Academy of Pediatrics recommends limiting screen use under two years, and then only for one hour tops for ages two to five. Limit device time and choose quality, slow-paced games and programs, From day 1, make a rule that all devices stay out of bedrooms at night and are turned off one to two hours before bedtime.

- **Make bedtime less of a battle.** Kiddos rarely want to stop playing to go to bed, so make that easier by giving them a five- or ten-minute heads-up (you can even set your smartphone). Also have a set lights-out time: if our daughter completes her bedtime routine before 8:15 P.M., she gets to read on her own, giving her incentive to cooperate.

- **Transitioning from crib to bed.** The day that baby starts climbing out of the crib feels a little tragic because now all bets are off. Don't feel the need to transition based just on age. Many children will stay in their crib as late as three. Also, try to avoid switching at a time of other major transitions, such as a new school or new baby if you can (instead, switch to the big-kid bed two or three months in advance). When that happens, allow your child to choose new linens for her new bed or even a new soft toy if she'd like, or let her stick to her old lovey if she prefers that familiarity.

- **Reinforce staying in bed.** Once your child is out of the crib, it's important to reinforce the rule that, after bedtime, you stay in bed unless necessary. If your child comes out of his room, gently walk him back to bed. Resist the urge to play or tell stories, so there's little value to getting up.

- **Deal with "monster" fears.** Children start to develop fears of the dark as well as nightmares and night terrors at this age. Acknowledge these fears and encourage your child. We keep a squirt bottle of "monster repellant spray" (water) that we mist "for protection" when needed. Dr. Altmann says, "I leave kisses on their pillow, in case they wake up and need kisses to get back to sleep." If your child is having nightmares or night terrors, look for potential contributors, such as being overtired (night terrors are more likely when a child's exhausted) or seeing violent or frightening TV shows, movies, or video games. If nightmares or night terrors persist, talk to your pediatrician.

PART 4
Resilience

187

Nurture the Relationships that Nourish You

Wednesday, March 14: I'm trying not to cry in front of an electrician in my living room.

My one-year-old had recently contracted norovirus and ended up in the ER.

A flood in our house meant we had to move out for two weeks (which occurred while I was live on-air and my cameraman held up a *Say Anything*–style sign: "NANNY CALLED. FIRE ALARM GOING OFF. FLOOD. EVERYONE OK, CALL IMMEDIATELY." *And now for a word from our sponsors . . .*).

A family member had just received very bad health news.

I was behind on my book manuscript—namely the "Resilience" section, *which is pretty twisted humor on your part, Universe.*

And my babysitter called out sick . . . for the entire week.

And just like that, my plans, backup plans, and backups for my backups collapsed.

Cue electrician with more flood-related concerns.

Some days as a mom, you swear you're being punk'd.

Of course, there are days when we have it together and everyone is fed and clean and deadlines are met. Then there are *those* days. Because between our children, work, and caring for our parents, motherhood today comes with many more expectations than a generation ago. Plus, landmark findings by Dr. Elissa Epel, UCSF Director of the Aging, Metabolism and Emotions Center, on stress and weight gain show that how we experience stress has even changed, creating a state of what I call the Chronic Stress Disequilibrium.[1]

Chronic Stress Disequilibrium

Here's how stress is supposed to work:

✓ Tiger jumps out at you from the jungle.

✓ You have an immediate stress response: adrenaline, cortisol, blood pressure, and heart rate increase to prepare you for "fight or flight."

✓ You fight or flee, and—assuming you don't get eaten Nat Geo–style—you get away.

✓ Now that you're safe, the stress response ends: hormones reset to normal, and you relax.

Except that's not how it happens today. Today, our stressors aren't tigers that we can escape. They're incessant: overwhelming demands on our time, financial concerns, a frustrating coworker, or 24/7 bad news on the TV. Problem is, your brain interprets it all the same way, mounting a stress response each time. That leaves us in a constant state of elevated stress and hypervigilance . . . and misery.

You know that stress makes you feel lousy, but chronically elevated stress does more harm than that. It affects the entire family, which is why, when Johnny starts acting up, the teacher will first quietly ask, "Is everything all right at home?" (*Would you like a side of mommy guilt with that stress?*) It also makes you physically ill, increasing your chances of getting a cold, having an accident, destabilizing your DNA (because, *science*), and even shortening your life span. Plus (no, I'm not done), the chronic stress disequilibrium causes a vicious cycle of cravings, weight gain, and constantly feeling depleted.

Do you feel that?

Enough. We can't always control the world around us, but we can take back this new world of mom-hood. We all have our equivalent of norovirus/flood/family-health-gate at one point or another, and I know this can help you get through yours. (In which case, all of those events actually improved this book because I needed to use every single hack for my own sanity.)

Remember: None of us get it right all the time. Forgive yourself. Your children do not need you to be perfect because having a perfect mother would be impossibly annoying and likely require years of very expensive therapy—so really, your imperfections are also *saving them money and they are welcome*. They simply need to see you react with love to them, to others, and—just as importantly—to yourself.

My Days Are a Blur

Hack 84
What's Your "Why"?

. . . and are you living by that? I'll admit—this hack goes deep. But I've seen too many ER patients only realize this at the end of their lives. Please don't wait. Live by it today. Let me share a story: on April 21, 2014, Rachel, one of my close friends since seventh grade, lost her children, Reagan and Jax, and mother in one devastating instant. She could have let that define her and shut down completely—no one would have blamed her. Except she didn't. Here's what she told me:

> When it comes to coping afterward, I leaned on my faith. I pulled from a bucket that was constantly being filled my entire life. I face things head-on. I don't focus on the life or options that no longer exist. I don't like to wallow or let my entire life be defined by grief. Nothing about Reagan and Jax was full of sadness or self-pity. *The only way to keep their lights shining is to live how they would here on earth and how I know they are in heaven.*

Rachel honors Reagan and Jax every day—and the Reagan and Jax Cohen Memorial Fund has raised $1 million for children's charities [1]. She's also had two more beautiful babies, Bo and Larkin. I don't share this as some sad, cautionary tale—it's not in some "Life is hard" section—that's not the point. It's about the *power* of living a life defined by what gives you meaning, and refusing—as Rachel does every day—to take your eyes off that. That's what leads people to make health changes (which is why people with a strong sense of meaning live longer lives[2]). It enables us to move mountains. It brings the beautiful in this at-times brutal world: your "hidden treasure in the darkness" (Isaiah 45:23). It's what gives us strength and bravery we never knew we had.

But in the busy-ness of our lives, it can be easy to overlook, like my ER patients sometimes have done. Please don't. Later, we'll cover how to find time to prioritize your "Why" (because let's face it, dishes still need to be done and bills paid). For now, I just want you to identify and write it down. That act alone can remind me of the abundance I take for granted, and also where I need to focus.

Chase the dream. Love on your children. Lean into your faith. Live by whatever is most important to you.

Because there is no dry run. There are no do-overs.

So let me ask you: How do *you* want to define your big, messy, *beautiful*, blessing of Life?

- **Name your primary "Why".** What takes your breath away and makes your life *rich*? This can include children, your faith, career, or a specific cause (or all of the above).

- _____

- _____

- _____

- **Identify some secondary "Why".** What smaller things fuel you? Maybe you sing, play an instrument, or dance. Maybe you volunteer, have an inner artist, or love to discover new cultures.

- _____

- _____

- _____

Hack 85
Live by Your "Why"

Steven Covey shared the following story in his book, *First Things First:*[3]

[The instructor] reached under the table and pulled out a wide-mouth gallon jar. He set it on the table next to a platter with some fist-sized rocks on it. "How many of these rocks do you think we can get in the jar?" he asked.

After we made our guess, he said, "Okay. Let's find out." He set one rock in the jar . . . then another . . . then another. I don't remember how many he got in, but he got the jar full. Then he asked, "Is that jar full?"

Everybody looked at the rocks and said, "Yes."

Then he said, "Ahhh." He reached under the table and pulled out a bucket of gravel. Then he dumped some gravel in and shook the jar and the gravel went in all the little spaces left by the big rocks. Then he grinned and said once more, "Is the jar full?"

By this time we were on to him. "Probably not," we said.

"Good!" he replied. And he reached under the table and brought out a bucket of sand. He started dumping the sand in and it went in all the little spaces left by the rocks and the gravel. Once more he looked at us and said, "Is the jar full?"

"No!" we all roared.

He said, "Good!" and he grabbed a pitcher of water and began to pour it in. He got something like a quart of water in that jar. Then he said, "Well, what's the point?"

Somebody said, "Well, there are gaps, and if you really work at it, you can always fit more into your life."

"No," he said. "That's not the point. The point is this: if you hadn't put these big rocks in first, would you ever have gotten any of them in?"

The big rocks are your primary "why," the pebbles your secondary ones. The sand and water are those things that simply take our time. When people describe their life as "crazy," their problem isn't too many big rocks. The problem is that they're filling their life jar with sand and water first. Their jars and schedule are full, but their hearts are not.

- **Prioritize your "why" activities.** To create space for your "why," you first have to take out some of the sand and water, so I give you permission to say "no" to some activities. Actually, it's doctor's orders. Then, once you've cleared out space, find ways to nurture your "why" every day. That doesn't mean you have to ditch your responsibilities and run away with the circus—even small amounts of time are soul nurturing. Take ten minutes to really listen to and connect with your child. To work on that side hustle you love or to engage in that hobby that just makes you feel *human* again.

- **Look for the "EEEEE!" that "why" brings.** One of my best college girlfriends and I labeled moments of unbridled joy as "EEEEE!": you got an A on that impossible assignment, your crush called you, you got front-row seats to the Indigo Girls ("*the closer I am to fi-iiine*"). We've grown up a little bit, and what triggers EEEEE! has changed, but the feeling is the same. Now, EEEEE! might come from landing a big client or deal, getting a "Mommy, you're my favorite lovey," or scoring tickets to Bruce Springsteen (*Bruuuuuuce!!*). These feelings aren't just fun; they're a barometer of how you're prioritizing your "why," which means that if you're not getting them, you may need a little more "why" activity in your life.

- **Take extra time to savor the** EEEEE! Research shows that intentionally acknowledging and savoring positive moments daily, boosts happiness in as little as a week. Sometimes EEEEE! moments are obvious; other times it may just feel like a warmth in your chest or a subtle tingling feeling that you could easily miss. Start to "listen" for that feeling and relish it when you notice it. Actually say "EEEEE!" if you want! (my daughter and I certainly do).

Hack 86
Start Your Day with Intention

What's your first thought when you wake up? If it's "Darn alarm!" or "I have *so* much to do today," that initial frustration and anxiety sets your focus for the entire day.

By default, our brain is evolutionarily wired to fixate on threats (more on this later). That means that when you wake up, your mind will habitually go to what could go wrong that day—unless you deliberately override it. By *intentionally* focusing on something positive, you can redirect your brain—and your entire day.

- **Start your day with a quick mantra.** Behavioral psychologist B. J. Fogg starts his day with "It's gonna be a great day." Gabrielle Bernstein suggests several in *May Cause Miracles*, such as "I am grateful for what I have, and I welcome all the gifts this day will bring." Our brain is constantly evolving, and the more you focus on a specific thought, be it positive or negative, the more you incorporate it into your subconscious and future thoughts. Put up a sticky note with the mantra, so you remember to say it first thing.

- **Be selective in how you wake up.** If you wake up to an alarm that sounds like an air raid, you're flooded with adrenaline before you even open your eyes. (Unless there *actually is* an air raid, I see no purpose in starting your day thinking so.) Instead, consider a favorite song, or at least a quieter alarm tone. Wake up to the sun (if it's light before you wake up) or a light-up alarm clock.

- **Connect with your partner.** Research has shown that taking fifteen seconds to turn toward each other, make eye contact, and say an affectionate "good morning" anchors your connection and interactions with each other all day.

- **Begin with a sun salutation.** A sun salutation is a wonderful yoga sequence to shake off the sleep and energize. Find my routine online at www.drdarria.com/momhacks (password: unstoppable), which consists of (1) stand straight and reach to the sky, (2) bend over and let your weight pull your hands to the floor, (3) step into plank, (4) move to cobra pose, (5) downward dog, (6) jump your feet to your hands, (7) then slowly stand back up.

- **Do routine activities the night before.** As much as possible, take care of the mundane the night before to make your morning less stressful. That includes making lunches, pulling out frozen meat to thaw in the fridge, and setting out the kids' school clothes.

Hack 87
Practice Gratitude—All Day

When I moved into my first home after college, I was so excited. I had my own washer and dryer that didn't require quarters or an ID! I had my own kitchen with a real oven instead of a toaster, and even my own bathroom. I felt awash in luxury. Well, at least for a few months. Soon, the kitchen began to feel small and dated (and not just because a fondue-party fiasco left my kitchen smelling like grilled cheese for life). I wanted a bathroom with a bathtub. What had once seemed luxurious quickly became not enough.

Significant positive changes transiently increase our happiness, but over the long term, we reset our expectations and revert to our prior level of happiness (known as our Happiness Set Point). That's why lottery winners aren't happier than anyone else; after their initial burst of euphoria, they eventually settle back to their happiness set point.

Psychologists call this cycle the "Hedonic Treadmill," and the way to beat it is not by running faster after our ever-expanding expectations, but by changing your Happiness Set Point. To change your Happiness Set Point you don't need more *stuff*; instead, you change it by building *gratitude* for what you do have.

Studies show that people who habitually express gratitude are more likely to be compassionate, happier, and healthier. Children with greater gratitude also perform better in school and have better social support.

- **Find gratitude in the mundane.** Look for opportunities for gratitude everywhere: that no one in your household has an ear infection *today,* that with the click of an app, toilet paper *shows up* at your door, that you know where your next meal is coming from. Albert Einstein famously said, "There are only two ways to live your life: as if nothing is a miracle, or as though everything is."

- **Encourage your children to voice gratitude.** Research has shown that, for adolescents, something as simple as "counting your blessings" was linked with more optimism and life satisfaction.[4] Play a round of "roses and thorns" at dinner, or simply ask your child to name something for which she is grateful during her bedtime routine.

- **Write one thing for which you're grateful at night.** As part of your own bedtime routine, write one person/thing/event for which you're grateful. Be specific and choose something different nightly to widen your gaze to all the abundance we never even notice. When it's for people who are present, make a point of telling them, or if not, send them a text or e-mail.

Hack 88
Be Present Now

A coworker and I have a weekly Sunday check-in—and some weeks, that Sunday text leaves me wondering, "Where did another week go?" If you feel the same, you know that this is a life stage where family, work, and caring for older parents seem to all intersect. When every day feels like a rat race, we run through life rarely fully present in *anything*.

The solution is to intentionally bring your focus to the present to quiet the 24/7 distractions, the comparisons, the concerns and allow the good to register. A Hebrew prayer reminds us, "Days pass, and the years vanish, and we walk sightless among the miracles."[5] Mindfulness is linked to improved attention and working memory, less depression, better relationship[6] and life satisfaction,[7] vitality, and fulfilment.[8] *Sign me up.*

Your Brain Is Wired to Always Be Looking Around

Our brain is wired for distraction: it's constantly scanning our environment, looking for threats, questioning the past, looking to the future. But that protective tendency can keep us so caught up in these internal dialogues that we miss the present moment (especially with the many distractions available to us today, thanks to our smartphones).

I used to think that if I wasn't constantly focusing on the next goal, I'd fail. I confused appreciation of the current moment with complacency, when, in fact, it's the fire that fuels creativity and success. It's okay to work to change a situation. But, in the meantime, find happiness where you are today. *Embracing the joy you can have in the present is the only way to create a tomorrow that you love.*

- **See the forest—and the beauty.** When people rehash the trite phrase "enjoy this time," I'd like to offer to let them stay up with the baby at night. But I now believe that what they mean (whether they realize it or not) is not so much "enjoyment" as *presence*. Remember that unless we intentionally override it, our brain is wired to focus on the negative and threats. I noticed this the other day when I was hiking with my family—I was focused on watching for snakes, swatting away spiders, and making sure my daughter didn't step in poison ivy, and I never looked up and just took a breath. In fact, it wasn't until I could see the clearing at the end of our hike that I realized I had missed out on enjoying the whole thing. I had literally missed the forest for the trees. "Enjoy this time" doesn't mean that you enjoy the snakes, ticks, and poison ivy (or dirty diapers, exhaustion, and tantrums), but that you can still have moments to notice the beauty all around you as well.

- **Do a mindfulness kick start to shut down the distractions.**
  - **Mini-mindfulness exercise.** Identify an object (ideally something natural, such as a flower or tree). Set your phone timer for one minute. Look at the object as if it's the first time you're seeing it. If it's a flower, what color is it? Are all the petals the same color? Do any look discolored or uneven? Can you smell it? Is it moving in the wind? See how many things you can observe in that time. After you've done this a few times, you can expand the exercise to two to five minutes.
  - **Guidance for a mindfulness meditation.** Do an online mindfulness meditation (UCLA Mindfulness Awareness Research Center[9] and Jeremy Hunter[10] both have free sessions of three to five minutes), or download an app such as Headspace or Simple Habit.

- **Start with short intervals of presence.** We won't break our distraction habit overnight. So, after doing one of the mindfulness kick-start exercises, aim for five minutes of being singularly present with a family member, without distraction from your phone or other to-dos. Slowly increase the time, and feel the difference in your interactions. You may even notice that your memory of these interactions improves because you're fully present.

Hack 89
Stop Multitasking

We think we are good multitaskers. We are not. In fact, neuro-science shows that we really don't *multi*task, we simply switch back and forth between tasks, with each switch burning brain glucose, losing attention, and increasing cortisol levels.[11] It also sucks time: shifting from one task to read an e-mail, for instance, requires fifteen minutes to get back into the first task, lowers productivity by up to 40 percent, doubles your rate of error, and diminishes memory. Bottom line is that *you don't have time to multitask.*

Not only that, if you're trying to multitask while engaging with someone else, it shows. Your kids don't know that you're looking at your phone because you're ordering items for them or because your impossible boss is demanding a response. They just presume that they're not worth your attention at that moment—not what you intend.

- **Single-tasking.** Instead of trying to play with your kids *and* order sippy cups from Amazon, *and* send that work reply e-mail, play with your kids, *then* order from Amazon, *then* reply. It may sound like it takes more time, but the increased efficiency of single-task focus will more than make up for it. Plus, you'll avoid ordering twelve bottles of your husband's shampoo because you were distracted (because I did that).

- **Compartmentalize.** Research shows that the most resilient people are able to compartmentalize well (hmmm . . . men may be onto something). Practice the mindfulness exercises to help close out distractions and compartmentalize.

- **Block time on your calendar.** If you have specific projects that have to be done, block out time to work on them. When I was writing this book, it led to a never-ending to-do list. So, instead of just trying to squeeze it in when I had a moment, I took the to-dos and blocked them out on the calendar, to make sure I'd have the time. Then make sure to single-task during each block.

- **Turn off devices and e-mail when you're working on a project.** Bill Gates goes on thinking retreats—just to think! Some executives only check e-mail during specific intervals. Studying the habits of these uber-successful individuals shows that they are not "always connected"—in fact, they intentionally disconnect.

Hack 90
Break the Device Habit

Do you pull out your device any time you have a quiet moment, whether it's just checking e-mail while the kids are playing or standing in line at the grocery store? The biggest enabler of our distraction habit is our smartphones.

In fact, recent research shows that our smartphones worsen our ability to focus,[12] increase our risk of an error or misinterpretation when we return to a task after using them, drive our attempts to multitask, and contribute to poorer working memory.[13]

- **Keep devices away from the meal table and family time.** Parents who use a smartphone at dinner are less likely to engage with their children, and those children are more likely to act out.[14] Another study showed that just the presence of smartphones harmed conversation and inter-personal connection.[15] Put away all devices during meal and family time to keep the focus on each other.

- **Allow for idle, quiet space, without pulling out your phone.** How many of us pull out the smartphone during any downtime, including going to the bathroom (*looks around, sheepishly raises hand*). Why are we so afraid of being with our thoughts that we can't pee in peace? For the next week, when you have a few idle moments, whether that's brushing your teeth, standing in line at the grocery store, or . . . yes . . . going to the bathroom, don't pick up your phone. You'd be surprised at how much brain space and creativity can open up when you're not so quick to fill it with distraction.

- **Don't rely on your smartphone.** Some scientists theo-rize that smartphones harm our memory because we get lazy—and assume we don't have to remember things be-cause we can always look them up. Periodically, try to re-member something without scribbling it in your phone or using GPS.

Cracking
Mommy Guilt and Self-Doubt

Hack 91
Ditch the Supermom Myth and
Accept Your Mom Evolution

According to Merriam-Webster's dictionary, the definition of "supermom" is "an exemplary mother; also: a woman who performs the traditional duties of housekeeping and child-rearing while also having a full-time job."

Bahahahahaahahaahaha . . . gasp . . . bahahahaah . . . wheeze. I mean, all we need is a cape!

Are they kidding? Did some 1950s ad-man write that? We have all shed tears when we've fallen short of our supermom goals—me included. Did none of us realize that we were crying about something as imaginary as leprechauns? Or the tooth fairy?

Before baby was born, we all had blissful visions of motherhood: days spent caressing our child, a golden aura around us like some picture from a Christmas pageant. As MTV's *Diary* series said, "You think you know, but you have no idea."

In reality, motherhood is a daily negotiation with chaos, both humbling and reaffirming. Some things are harder than we expected, while others come more naturally than we dared dream.

It does none of us any service to cling to this caricature of motherhood. In fact, trying to live up to this ideal only makes us feel inadequate and increases our risk for depression and anxiety.[1]

The only perfect parents are the ones who haven't had children yet.

Let's have a motherhood reset.

- **Recognize that you're evolving a new identity.** When baby is born, your identity changes, which means that the woman you spent decades becoming is suddenly slightly different. In a piece for the *New York Times*, Dr. Alexandra Sacks notes that anthropologists label this evolution *matrescence*[2] and liken it to the growing pains of adolescence: uncertainty, acne, hormone fluctuations, emotional roller coasters, and all. Your former self needn't disappear. You will again find time to exercise, talk to your spouse, create art, or lead companies or civic organizations, should you wish. Or you may do something else entirely. Give yourself the time and grace to evolve, and enjoy the woman who emerges.

- **Stop blaming yourself when events diverge from the fantasy.** I've seen many a new-mom-to-be frantic because a life-saving delivery did not match with her birth plan or because her experience nursing didn't match her expectations. I'm equally guilty: When I was thirty-seven weeks pregnant with my second child, I realized he had stopped moving; three hours later, I was in an emergency C-section. My baby was healthy and beautiful, and yet I was so busy blaming myself for the early delivery that I was missing the perfect tiny human before me. That's the problem with the fantasy: unmet expectations—no matter how ludicrous— are interpreted as failure, and fixating on what *isn't* can make us miss the beauty of what *is*.

- **Acknowledge your feelings without guilt.** Our feelings as mothers are complex. There are ups and downs, and no mother feels joy, love, and perfect peace toward her child at all times. As Dr. Sacks put it, "Most of the time, the experience of motherhood is not good *or* bad, it's both good *and* bad." You will ache for your child to just go to sleep. Then the minute he's in his crib, you'll want to hold him again. You'll crave personal time yet think of your child the entire time you're away. This is normal.

- **Stop the perfect mom s**t.** The pressure to be a perfect mom can take the fun out of mom-ing (and out of being a kid, too). So, reality reset: Your kids do *not* care if their lunchbox food is carved into stars. Your newborn nursery needn't look like Jessica Alba's. When *we* were babies, our "nurseries" looked like the rest of the house (which at my house was orange and brown shag rugs). We were *babies* and did not care. Your kids don't need mommy perfection as proof of your love. They need you just as you are, loving-to-the-moon-and-back mom, warts and all.

Hack 92
Choose Your Thoughts

The Buddha once said, "We are what we think. All that we are arises with our thoughts. With our thoughts we make the world."

Our thoughts and emotions are creations of our brain. Maybe you're thinking, "That sounds pretty new agey. . . . I thought this woman was a *medical doctor*. . . . " But go with me. We take our thoughts and emotions as truth. But what if they're not? What if they're more a result of our interpretations?

Don't believe me?

Well, did you hear a Yanni or a Laurel?

Was it a blue dress or a gold dress?

See what I mean? Our subconscious brain takes in millions of bits of information in a second—but our conscious brain can only process a fraction of that. So our subconscious brain determines what gets through to conscious thought. That leaves a lot of room for interpretation—and error.

That's how one person can walk through Manhattan and see exciting activity and shopping and the bright lights of Broadway, and another come away commenting on the smells, the garbage, the crowds, and the noise.

The science is clear: our thoughts and emotions are affected less by our *circumstances* and more by where we focus our *attention* and *interpretation*. In a study by positive psychologists Ed Diener and Martin E. P. Seligman of more than two hundred undergraduates, they found sharp differences in levels of happiness—but no connection between happiness and life experiences. In fact, students in the top 10 percent for happiness had the same number of positive life experiences as those in the bottom 10 percent.[3]

It isn't what happens to us that causes us to suffer; it's what we say to ourselves about what happens.

—Pema Chodron

Primitive (Fast) Brain Versus
Wiser (Slow) Brain

For our earliest ancestors, the unknown could be deadly: an approaching tiger or an enemy warlord. The secret to survival was to assume the worst and ask questions later, a response driven by what researchers like Dr. Daniel Kahneman call the "fast brain."

Over millennia, our brains also developed the "slow brain," the prefrontal cortex (PFC), which holds our executive functioning and reasoning. Think of the PFC as Pinocchio's Jiminy Cricket (or David Spade, as I mentioned in the nutrition section): a wise, slower voice.

The fast brain reacts first, with a *Ready! Fire! . . . Aim!* mentality. By the time the slow brain chimes in with reason, the fast brain is already off to the races.

That evolutionary response was useful when any potential threat could be deadly, but when our threats are a tone-deaf e-mail, traffic, overpacked schedule, or potentially hurtful comment from our child or spouse, our automatic fight-or-flight response is counterproductive and exhausting. But, just like Pinocchio learned to listen to Jiminy Cricket, you can learn to listen for your slow brain by intentionally choosing your thoughts. As Amit Sood says in *The Mayo Clinic Guide to Stress-Free Living,* "When you choose your thoughts, you're more likely to think positively; random thoughts are more likely to be ruminative and negative."[4]

Automatic negative thoughts. Automatic negative thoughts (ANTs) are the outcome of your fast brain's quick response plus your brain's tendency to create habits. They occur when our fast brain jumps to conclusions, creating patterns that we reinforce every time we think them. They're our negative inner monologue on replay. Even though ANTs are more based on our insecurities than actual facts, we automatically believe them—unless we learn to challenge them.

So you can choose: Where do you focus your attention? It's simple driver's ed: if you suddenly see an obstacle in the road (such as a wooden box that fell off a truck), your brain's tendency is to fixate on the negative—in this case the box (see Primitive [Fast] Brain Versus Wiser [Slow] Brain). But driver's ed teaches us that, to avoid an accident, you must do exactly the opposite—you must override that tendency to stare at the box because you will drive right into where you're focusing your attention. Instead, you have to look where you want to drive. *Fixate not on the negative you want to avoid, but on where you want to go.*

NOTE: Read this hack and #93 for how to recognize ANTs, and #94 to learn to challenge them.

- **Learn to recognize your ANTs.** The key sign of an ANT is when you suddenly feel your mood shift negatively. Also, look for the following red flags:
  - Thoughts that include "always" or "never": A statement from your spouse triggers "He always criticizes me, our relationship will never work."
  - Black-and-white thinking: Feedback on your presentation leads to "My entire presentation was a disaster."
  - Mind reading: "They didn't say 'hi' to me this morning. They must be upset with me."
  - Catastrophizing: "I'm going to damage my relationship with my children. I'm an awful mom."

- **Remember that you can choose how you experience every single moment.** Julia Rogers Hamrick suggests using the phrase "I choose easy world" in her book, *Choosing Easy World*. It's not *Pollyanna*; it simply means that you're making the mental choice that when things get tough, you choose the drama-free interpretation. Try it the next time you start to get frustrated. It works.

Hack 93
Identify Your Inner Critic

For most of us, the strongest ANTs are those we direct internally, via our inner critic (IC). Of our 50,000 thoughts every single day, 80 percent of them are negative, with an average eight self-criticisms a day.[5]

Drs. Pauline Clance and Suzanne Imes coined the term "impostor phenomenon" after studying hundreds of successful women, and found, "Despite their earned degrees, . . . praise and professional recognition . . . these women do not experience an internal sense of success. They consider themselves to be 'impostors.'"[6]

Again, we believe what we tell ourselves. But your inner critic is nothing more than another ANT. She's not the truth. She's the mean girl who knows all your emotional buttons and goads you with them. In fact, if anyone actually verbalized what your IC says, you'd slap a restraining order on her. She wouldn't even be allowed on *Real Housewives,* which is why it's time to give her a good "girl, bye."

- **Recognize what your inner critic sounds like.** The IC is that nasty voice telling you that you're screwing up. You forgot your child's costume party and immediately think, "I'm a failure as a mom, and my child will never forgive me." When your outfit is a little too tight, you think, "I'm disgusting. I'll never lose weight." Your inner critic is a b***h; and she's not worth your time.

- **Label her.** To start, just label the voice. The next time you hear the IC, say internally or aloud, "That's my inner critic." That alone can remind you that it's not necessarily the truth.

- **Ask yourself whether would you want someone to talk to your child that way.** Even if we don't voice our inner critic's messages verbatim, our children can internalize them. The words we choose to describe ourselves today will be what our children someday use to describe themselves. If you wouldn't want your own daughter to believe it about herself someday, don't let yourself believe it now.

Hack 94
Challenge Your Automatic Negative Thoughts and Inner Critic

Once you've learned to identify your ANTs and inner critic, the next step is to challenge them. This is hard because ANTs create tunnel vision: they dominate your thoughts in a moment, making it increasingly difficult to see any good, discounting the positive, and causing catastrophizing.

- **Remind yourself that your ANTs are not truth.** Your ANTs are more like the result of playing the "telephone game" than a true reflection of reality. Simply ask, "Is that really true?" or tell yourself, "That's probably not even true" to just open the door for your slow brain to kick in.

- **Make a list of the good.** To counter phenomenon syndrome or the inner critic, keep a list of positive feedback or outcomes you had, so that the next time you're stuck in self-criticism mode and unable to see any of the good that you've done, it's right there in black and white.

- **Replace the ANT with truth.** Go through the table below paraphrased from *Mind over Mood*,[7] to identify your typical ANT, and find evidence against it. Keep it handy for the next time you're locked in ANT tunnel vision.

214

Ask Yourself the Following	Examples	Fill in Your Own
(1) Ask yourself: What event triggered this feeling?	*I forgot to send my daughter with a costume for her school activity.*	
(2) Then ask: What was the root cause/ catastrophic ANT that jumped into my mind?	*I'm an awful mother and my child will hate me. (Other common ANTs for different scenarios include "my marriage will fall apart, I'll lose my job, I'll never lose weight.")*	
(3) Challenge the ANT: *"Is this really true?"* or *"How likely is that really?"* Identify any facts to the contrary. Have you had experiences in the past to show that your ANT was *not* true? Are you discounting any facts that may disprove your ANT? Are you ignoring any successes/strengths or other assets you have shown?	*I'm usually really good at remembering most school activities. My daughter won't likely care about this single one, and another mom likely forgot it, too. I did that school event last week that made her so happy, so I had that mommy win.*	

Ask Yourself the Following	Examples	Fill in Your Own
(4) Replace your ANT with a more balanced thought. What would you tell your best friend if she felt that way? What would she tell you? What is really a more realistic outcome/interpretation of this event?	*Your daughter will be sad for about three minutes and forget as soon as it's snack time. You're a freaking amazing mom, and schools have too many events nowadays anyway. Whatever happened to just doing reading and math?*	

Hack 95
Recognize Baby Blues and Postpartum Depression

Our emotions can go haywire during pregnancy and the first postpartum year. In fact, 80 percent of moms experience what's called the "baby blues" (and the remaining 20 percent probably were too tired to answer the survey), with 10–15 percent of those experiencing postpartum depression (PPD).[8]

Yet, despite how common these feelings are, we bottle them up. So, let's clear the air: although there are certain risk factors for PPD (such as genetics and prior history[9]), it can happen to *anyone*. There is *no* connection with being a "good" or "bad" mom. In fact, if you talk about it, you're an amazing mom who is willing to be vulnerable for the sake of herself and her child. And that makes you brave. You would not hesitate to seek medical care if you had the flu; these feelings are no different.

- **Know the signs of baby blues.** Symptoms include crying for no apparent reason, mood swings, anxiety and irritability, and feeling overwhelmed. These symptoms pop up sporadically, are not constant, and typically go away on their own.

- **Know the signs of PPD.** Symptoms of PPD aren't sporadic and can occur almost constantly, on most days:
  - Depressed mood (being tearful, sad, empty, or hopeless)
  - Loss of interest or pleasure in most activities and people, including your baby
  - Insomnia or hypersomnia (needing too much sleep)
  - Constant fatigue or loss of energy
  - Feeling worthless or excessive guilt
  - Decreased ability to think or concentrate
  - Thoughts of death, harming yourself, or harming your baby
  - Seeming agitated/rushing/restless, or consistently slowed down to others

- **If you're feeling overwhelmed, put down the baby.** Sometimes, the baby won't stop crying, and you reach a breaking point. If you're alone and that happens, it's okay to put the baby into her crib safely and walk away for a moment. I'll never forget hearing this reassurance from Dr. William Sears, who acknowledged that every mom just needs a break sometimes.

- **This is me, asking you.** Studies show that unless a mother is questioned directly about these thoughts, she typically will not share them with anyone.[10] So, I'm asking you: Do you have these feelings? If so, please share them with someone you trust.

- **Reach out for support.** Without treatment, symptoms of PPD last up to a year and may be linked to development delays in the child. Call your ob-gyn, pediatrician, various postpartum help lines, or a crisis hotline. If you are truly at risk, go to the ER. Please, please do not try to handle frightening feelings alone.

- **Know that *many* treatment options exist.** Some women don't seek help because they think the only treatment is medication. Let me put that myth to rest. First-line treatments include many non-medication therapies. For women who need medications, your doctor can help choose one with you and baby both in mind.

If You're Feeling Overcommitted and Exhausted

Hack 96
Ask for Help

Regardless of our roles *outside* the home, most moms also carry most of the home-based responsibilities. If you feel like you're juggling too many things—and none of them well—it's time to call in reinforcements and not feel one darn ounce of guilt about it. The phrase "it takes a village" exists because it *does*.

I must fully acknowledge that I can't imagine keeping these little ones alive without the support of my generous, ever-patient husband, who is a true partner in every sense of the word. But, I know that many moms are raising kids on their own *and I think you are amazing*—and that at times, every single one of us needs an extra hand. (Or two. Or four.)

Remember, the only people who expect you to "do it all" are those masochists who came up with the definition of supermom, and I guarantee that they never changed a diaper.

- **Take advantage of every free resource possible.** Can your dry cleaner deliver? Can you put your usual grocery staples onto subscription (in which case you'll likely save

time *and* money)? Can you swap child minding with another mom in the neighborhood?

- **Trade with your partner.** Have your partner take care of
  the baby on alternating nights so you can get some rest.
  Or split responsibilities: one of my coworkers does the
  cooking, while her husband does dishes and bathes the
  kiddos.

- **Outsource what you can.** Can your babysitter prep dinner or at least pick up the toys? Maybe a neighborhood
  high schooler can lend a hand with errands for a small
  fee. Ask a close family member to take care of the baby at
  night or hire a night nurse if you can—even if it's just
  once a week.

Hack 97
Employ Instant Relaxation Techniques

Working in the ER, I cannot afford to let stress get the better of
me; not only does it cloud my thinking, I know that my mood
sets the tone for my patients and staff. Being a mom isn't much
different in that way.

I was once working an overnight shift in a small ER, when a
woman came in labor. She was going to deliver the baby here.
Now. And I was the only doctor. I quickly realized that the um-
bilical cord was wrapped several times around the baby's neck,
and if the mother started to panic, it could cost the baby's life.

I breathed. I focused on the baby and used my best (fake)
calm voice to tell the mom "You're doing *so well!* You've earned
a little break, so just relax for a minute" because I needed to buy
time, and I couldn't afford to have her panic. Alongside me was
our charge nurse, a wonderful ER veteran who quickly realized
what I was doing, and calmly went to the head of the bed to

reassure mom while my mind and hands went through every maneuver to free the baby.

We stayed calm. Mom stayed calm, I slipped off the cord, and a beautiful baby was born.

When you're under enormous pressure, the fight-or-flight stress response can be counterproductive, which is why it's crucial to know how to short-circuit it.

- **Focus only on what needs to be done next.** The complexity of an ER trauma can be overwhelming, so we combat that by following the ABCs (airway, breathing, circulation). You can do the same—just focus on the *next* thing that needs to be done *right now*.

- **Quick breathing exercise.** Inhale for four beats, hold it for four beats, then let it out for four beats. If you can, pull your fingers into soft fists with each inhale, and relax them on exhale. Do this exercise five times.

- **Alternate nostril breathing.** Sitting quietly, use your index finger to block your left nostril. Inhale through your right nostril. Holding your breath, move your index finger to block your right nostril. Exhale through your left nostril, then inhale through your left nostril, hold your breath, and switch to unblock the right nostril/block the left nostril. Repeat this exercise for one or two minutes or until you start to feel more at ease.

- **Step outside.** Even a short walk can lower stress and anxiety. Not only that, taking a walk is a great way to exit a situation that's becoming increasingly tense. Go outside to get the added energizing effect of sunshine. Observe your surroundings, breathe deeply, and get out of your head.

- **Turn up the music and dance.** Listening to music reduces frustration and anxiety. Dance if you can, as dancing activates so many different brain regions that it's practically impossible to hold onto frustration.[1] Dancing can also improve cognitive function, which will help you better problem-solve.

- **Create a laugh list.** I have a list of things that make me laugh: my infant photo-bombing a video of my daughter singing, any *Carpool Karaoke* clip, and a few of my favorite comedians on Twitter. Whenever I need a quick pick-me-up, I know exactly where to go.

Hack 98
Employ Instant De-Angering Techniques

Today's world is full of big tempers, short fuses, and civility run amok. Turn on any *Real Housewives* episode (or drive the Atlanta perimeter highway) if you need proof.

Of course, when we're constantly under stress, our fuses become shorter. In these moments, lowering our stress levels isn't enough; we need tools to avoid saying anything we'll regret.

- **Buy yourself time.** The fast brain has you lashing out before you've even realized what's happened. In these moments, simply say, "I need some time" to buy yourself space to restrain your fast-brain response and give your slow brain time to weigh in.

- **Will it bother you in five years?** In half a decade, will you give a s**t? If not, then it doesn't matter now.

- **Assume positive intent.** Former PepsiCo CEO Indra Nooyi shared her father's advice: "Assume positive intent."[2] Imagine that you're driving down the highway and the car beside you suddenly swerves into your lane. Then it swerves into another lane, maniacally exiting the highway. Your first response: "@!*#&@*%#&%^#&!" But what if I told you that the driver of that car was a mom, whose baby was choking in the backseat? That changes things, doesn't it? The truth is, we never really know someone's intentions. If we start with a positive assumption, we create room to understand others—and keep our own anger at bay, regardless of their motivations.

- **See the context through the action.** We often veil vulnerability and hurt in anger: A daughter's "I don't love you" may actually stem from sadness that you're paying more attention to her brother. Instead of meeting her anger with your own, try to look for a source of pain behind the action. By focusing your attention there, your body releases oxytocin, which makes it easier to respond with empathy.[3] Yes, it is hard to *not* take the bait. But if you can see struggle beneath, you can respond to *that,* and not to the hurtful action.

- **Repeat a mantra or prayer.** Sometimes I repeat, "I have a lesson that I must learn here," or I follow Gabrielle Bernstein's advice in *May Cause Miracles* and simply repeat, "I choose to see them with love."[4] Let's be honest—the prayer is as much for ourselves as it is for the recipient.

Hack 99
Be in Nature

Hugged a tree recently? You should. According to the Nature Conservancy, children today get half as much outdoors time as the previous generation,[5] and we adults get even less.

Exposure to nature and sunlight is so *good* for us, whether we're walking in the woods, sitting on a bench in a park, or just looking at trees. Japanese researchers call this "forest bathing," and studies have found that it improves heart rate, blood pressure, and cortisol, lowers anger, and even boosts key immune cell functions.[6]

Getting more sunlight in the fall may help you fight off the flu that winter.[7] Plus, hospital patients who had views of trees from their hospital window (as opposed to a brick wall) healed more quickly in one study. So, the next time you're looking for a family activity, opt for a little "vitamin N" (nature, of course!).

- **Walk in a park or your neighborhood.** You needn't go to the Grand Tetons. A five- to ten-minute walk in a nearby park or local tree-lined neighborhood is beneficial.

- **Take a family or group hike.** In my family, we take a one-hour hike together every weekend. Search your city and "hiking trails" to find new places to explore.

- **Schedule daily outside time.** We have a routine that we go outside to play for fifteen to thirty minutes before dinner every night. Play catch, tag, or hide-and-seek or even just play with playdough or paint outside. And the next time you find yourself with a half hour with the kiddos, take it outdoors.

- **Have dinner al fresco.** Whether it's a workday lunch or family dinner, the outdoor setting boosts your mood, lowers stress levels, and even improves concentration. Besides, when you're outside, who cares how much food your toddler throws on the floor?

- **Activate your senses when you're outdoors.** What do you hear? Feel? See? Don't just pass by so quickly that you miss the leaves for the trees. Take this time to be present and savor your surroundings.

Hack 100
Eat for Your Brain

Our brains make up 2 percent of our body weight, yet they consume approximately 20 percent of our total energy. In addition, 90 percent of serotonin, one of the "happy" neurotransmitters, is made in the gut and is directly influenced by our microbiome and diet.

Unfortunately, today's Western diet increases our risk of depression by up to 30 percent compared to those on a Mediterranean-type diet.[8] Your child's mental health will be affected by his own diet, as well as what you ate in pregnancy[9] (for more see the "Nutrition" section).

- **Minimize sugar and processed grains.** In a study of people with depression, those put on a twelve-week Mediterranean-style diet with minimal processed grains were four times more likely to experience remission of their depression.[10]

- **Eat your omegas.** Fatty acid omega 3s, particularly DHA, are crucial for cognitive function and mood. But most of us (particularly women who are pregnant or just had a child) don't get enough. Find omega 3s in fatty fish, olive oil, tree nuts, flax seeds, and avocados. For pregnant and nursing women, doctors may recommend a DHA supplement.

- **Eat your fruits and veggies.** Mom was right. People who eat more produce, even after adjusting for demographics and lifestyle factors, feel less psychological distress and better mental health.[11] Research from New Zealand suggests that the impact can be felt in as little as two weeks.[12] Aim for five servings of produce daily, incorporating leafy greens and cruciferous vegetables with high amounts of vitamin C, vitamin A, sulforaphane, and folate.

- **Add fermented foods.** Early studies suggest that probiotics may also help improve anxiety levels and stress.[13] Good sources of probiotics include raw sauerkraut, kefir, yogurt, miso, and tempeh, among many others.

- **Check your levels.** If you're eating a good diet and still feeling stressed, talk to your doctor about checking your levels for vitamin D, vitamin B6, magnesium, folic acid, iron, and other vitamins and minerals. Although it's clear that it's better to get these nutrients in your food, a supplement can be beneficial when levels are too low.

Hack 101
Exercise for Your Brain

If I wanted to give you a magic pill for stress and anxiety, it would be exercise. People who exercise regularly show less overall vulnerability to stress[14] in as little as four weeks after starting the exercise habit.[15]

Exercise helps regulate anger after a stressful event,[16] improves your mood, enhances motivation and willpower, and even enhances mental alertness.[17] In a Duke University study of participants with major depression, regular exercise was as effective as taking a prescription antidepression medication.[18]

- **Even a short session helps mood.** Exercising one hour a week is linked with a 44 percent lower risk of depression.[19] As little as ten minutes can improve your immediate mood, according to one study,[20] and another found that riding an exercise bike for twenty minutes before giving a stressful speech lowered the stress response.[21]

- **What's the best exercise for stress?** Most important is that you choose what you like: when people choose their preferred exercise themselves, they get an additional mood boost and anxiety reduction, as opposed to those who do an exercise they are prescribed.[22] So stop doing exercises that you hate, and instead find something that fits your personality and that you enjoy.

- **Just** *move*. Particularly on those days that you can't fit in exercise, simply making an effort to get in more leisurely or general activity can boost your mood.[23] Whether it's a brisk walk, stretching at your desk, or calf raises outside your car before carpool, the less time you spend sitting, the better your mental health.

Hack 102
Start a Meditation or Prayer Habit

What happens when you put the Dalai Lama in an MRI?

No really, it's not a joke. In an effort to understand how meditation affects the brain, researchers at MIT teamed up with the Dalai Lama and other Buddhist monks to study the brains of frequent meditators,[24] and they found that meditation had the power to actually modify your brain.

But even more interesting were the results when they studied meditation novices, people like you and me. After an eight-week course, participants had persistent emotional benefits months later. Particularly beneficial for those of us with a short temper, they also had decreased the density of their fast brain (the amygdala).[25]

Prayer and meditation also evoke the relaxation response, lowering blood pressure and heart rate and even increasing life span.

Note for the skeptical: If you don't feel ready to take up meditation regularly, I absolutely understand. In that case, just try a two- or three-minute meditation a few times (Deepak Chopra has a few), the next time you're feeling stressed.

- **Just start.** When I thought I needed a "practice" of meditation, it sounded like work. All you need is a quiet spot and if you're new to it, a guided meditation. Choose one based on length of time (they can range from a super-short two minutes to thirty minutes or longer) and style (if one practitioner leaves you feeling antsy and watching the clock, try another). I like Gabrielle Bernstein, Deepak Chopra, Pema Chodron, Sadhguru Jaggi Vasudev (whose meditations tend to be long but energizing), Vedic meditation (if you dread sitting still), or apps like Headspace, or Simple Habit.

- **Pray.** Research shows the mental and physiological benefit of prayer, particularly when we pray for others. Also a prayer before a challenging event can help us persevere.[26]

- **Whenever you have a few empty minutes, use the time to meditate or pray.** It can be hard to find solid chunks of time when you have small children. Steal time for what I call "micro-meditations" or "micro-prayers." Whether you're waiting on hold, in the carpool line, or even at the post office, resist the urge to pull out your phone. Instead, close your eyes (if you can). Breathe in and feel the air enter, and breathe out. Envision sending your breath to any tense body parts and sending out the tension with every exhalation. Say a prayer if you wish. You'll feel a noticeable difference—and never see waiting in line the same way.

Nurture the Relationships
that Nourish You

Hack 103
Make Loved Ones Feel Like Rock Stars

I see it every time, no matter what the emergency. If someone else has brought a child to the ER, then when the child's mother arrives, her reaction is universal: every mama runs into that room, cradles her child to her chest, nestling their faces together.

"I love you" is what she says, while they embrace.

No one checks social media. No one is distracted by the day's to-dos.

I know that we can't live our lives in these little bubbles, but it does make me wonder—why don't we do it more often?

It shouldn't be surprising: Duke University research demonstrates that children who receive more affection and attention from their mothers experience less stress and anxiety and have better social interactions. Positive attention such as smiling, making eye contact, encouraging, and being physically loving can all boost your child's self-image and sense of security.

In the busyness of our daily lives, it's easy to take them for granted, running out of the house with only a cursory wave or kiss, picking up our children without getting off the phone.

For the next week, let's try to be extravagant with our love. *While you're at it, do the same for your partner, who often gets left out these days.*

- **Center yourself before you greet your family.** We bring home a lot of baggage that distracts us long after we walk in the door. Before you greet your family, do a mini–mindfulness exercise (see hack #88). Focusing your attention on something neutral helps you turn your attention away from frustrations, so you can turn it to your loved ones.

- **Greet your family like you haven't seen them in ages.** In *The Mayo Clinic Guide to Stress-Free Living,* Dr. Amit Sood asks, "Can you greet your loved ones at the end of each day as if you're seeing them for the first time after 10 days?" Just try it.

- **Compliment them.** Tell your children and partner that you love them and are proud of their hard work. Tell them that you're grateful for them, or that you respect their good behavior and support. Be as specific as possible, as frequently as you can.

- **Ask for their input.** A key piece of advice I've heard from many uber-successful moms is to treat the family calendar like a family decision, including activities, what you attend, and other family to-dos. Can't make the school parade *and* the after-school soccer game? Ask your child; he or she may not care about one, while the other matters greatly. When kids know that they have a say in your priorities, they better understand those times when conflicts arise.

- **Say yes when you can.** To the fast brain, saying no is the safer, easier decision, particularly if the request breaks a routine. Which is why when it's bedtime and your child asks for you to play with him for five minutes, or your spouse asks you to sit down and catch up when you have work to do, the knee-jerk reaction is "no." But life and memories are made in the fun in these unexpected moments. "No" may be easier and time-saving, but "yes" is what feeds your soul.

Hack 104
Connect with Your Partner

Do you feel like you and your partner started out like Prince Harry and Meghan, but now are closer to Al and Peggy Bundy? Your former deep soul-gazing conversations have been replaced by tag teaming diaper blowouts and catching up on work and TV after the kiddos go to bed.

It's not just nice to have; a loving relationship supports your mental health, reduces your risk of heart disease,[1] and even lengthens your life span. If you swore you'd never become one of "those" couples who lose touch . . . but have become one of "those couples," it may be time for a little connection reset.

- **Turn off your critical voice.** He didn't take out the garbage, didn't clean the kitchen, or just doesn't listen. Routine criticism leads to defensiveness, stonewalling, and contempt, which researchers John and Julie Gottmann characterize as the "four horsemen" that doom a relationship.[2] Before you say anything at all, first see whether you can envision his way as simply *different*, rather than *wrong*. I have a girlfriend whom I try to emulate—when her husband does something entirely differently than her perfectionist self would, she holds her tongue when she can. If you really do need to voice your concern (but honestly—*do you?*), keep it neutral and against the specific *behavior* (such as his chaotic bedtime routine), as opposed to an attack on your spouse as a parent.

- **Appreciate your spouse's efforts.** When I first met a good friend of my husband's, I was surprised to see how often he and his wife expressed gratitude to each other. I realized that it wasn't superfluous; it was smart. We all need to hear validation. Studies demonstrate that people who thank their partners for even the smallest things have more connection and satisfaction.[3]

- **Put away your phone when you're together.** When we're talking to people and they are looking at their phones, it makes us feel unimportant. Make a point of setting aside devices when you're having a conversation.

- **Do a weekly "board meeting" with your partner.** A good girlfriend started doing this with her husband every Sunday, at a time when they were feeling disconnected. After the kiddos are in bed, they each share six things for which they're thankful. They then go over the calendar for the week, and end with six dreams that they each have. No judgments allowed—just free space to share their wishes and goals. She told me that "it created an intimacy for us after nine years of marriage that we didn't even realize we were craving."

- **Share your plans.** Nothing is more disheartening than being vulnerable and having the other person reject or simply not notice it. If you choose to do a relationship hack, share those plans with your spouse. At a minimum, he'll be more likely to notice and appreciate any small changes— and perhaps even try to implement a few, as well.

Hack 105
Prioritize Intimacy

I was scrolling through a Facebook mom group when a post caught my eye. Another mom was concerned about the sex-related dreams she was having, despite the fact that she and her husband had sex three or four times a week, each with multiple orgasms. *Wait. Go back.* I love my dear fellow moms who responded with everything from, "Are you a fake Russian bot?" to "I got exhausted just reading this." If you're feeling that your friskiness has fizzled, that's normal.

- **Tease.** It takes no time to appreciatively slap your spouse's butt or to walk too closely and graze his front with your behind. Send a flirty text (just keep it in code, or risk explaining "sexy time" to your five-year old who just learned to read). If you have the opportunity and it crosses your mind, do it.

- **Cuddle.** Take time daily (or weekly) to physically connect, without any expectation of sex. Simply enjoy sharing each other's space.

- **Do "appreciations."** This one comes from tantric practices (yes, the kind Sting does, and I'm pretty sure he has sex seventy times a day) and was shared with me by San Francisco–based therapist Yael Melamed. For five minutes, face your partner, knees and hands lightly touching. Take turns saying one thing that you appreciate about the other, including physical "assets" as well as emotional and supportive ones.

- **Schedule sex.** I know. There's no way that Carrie and Big, or Princess Leia and Han Solo scheduled sex, right? They also never changed a blowout diaper or had to wear postpartum underwear, so there's that. According to experts (*I've always been curious about people who decide to specialize in sex research*), if we wait until we're ready for sex, we'll never have sex. In fact, scheduling sex weekly is linked with better relationship satisfaction. As Kelly Ripa puts it, "I fundamentally believe that the more you do it, the more you do it, the less you do it, the less you do it."[4] So, go ahead, create a little naughty appointment in your calendar (and just like the naughty texts, keep it in code).

Hack 106
Turn Toward Bids for Connection

Your spouse tries to embrace, but you brush him off while you're doing dishes. Or your child wants to play, but you're busy sending an e-mail. Dr. Richard Kannwischer, head pastor at Peachtree Presbyterian Church, taught what researcher John Gottman calls "bids for connection": tiny, subtle invitations to engage. In healthy relationships, 82 percent of bids are acknowledged, while it's only 19 percent in unhealthy ones.

John Ortberg suggests, "Each connection is like a deposit into an emotional bank account . . . when invitations are not recognized or embraced, relationships tend to die." The more we respond to bids, the more our trust and connections deepen—and beget more bids. On the flip side, if we don't notice them, the person sending out the bid is less likely to try again. Keep your relationship bank accounts growing by noticing and responding to bids as often as you can.

- **Listen for them.** We're often so caught up in our own worlds that we miss bids. Put away your devices, and remember that bids are subtle. They can be a smile or wink, a request for advice, an invitation to read a bedtime book or watch a video together, or even a moment to commiserate about a struggle.

- **How to say yes when it's inconvenient.** To meet a bid, you must respond on the requestor's time line, not yours. Which means it's not always convenient. Say yes if you can stop what you're doing. But if you can't, a loving response will still nurture the relationship. Instead of a distracted "I'm busy," try, "I love playing with you and I wish I could right now. I have to finish one thing. Can we promise to play in thirty minutes?"

- **Don't lash out if your own bids are ignored.** It hurts when someone neglects our bid, and our innate response is to cause hurt in return. Never, ever does that help. Calmly restate your need directly, such as "I'm trying to spend time with you," or even a simple "Ouch" or "That hurt my feelings." Most likely your child or spouse didn't realize you were trying to make a connection, and a neutrally repeated request will achieve the connection you're craving far better than a retaliatory response.

Hack 107
Love Your Village

Twenty years ago, the average American had three best friends, today we average one to two.

That's a shame because not only is it so much fun to see your BFs, they are key to your health. Having a strong, committed social network is key to longevity, boosting life span up to 50 percent. Also, having strong relationships takes pressure off your romantic partner to fulfill your every emotional need.

- **Schedule activities together that can include your kids.** Want to see your girlfriend who has children of the same age? Playdate! Go to the park, a walk, or just each other's houses.

- **Trade childcare with your spouse.** Every other Tuesday, one of my girlfriends and her husband alternate taking childcare duty so the other can go out with a buddy. They both get adult time, and the kiddos love the "special parent nights" as well.

- **Just schedule it.** Once every two months, have a standing date with your girlfriends. It doesn't have to be formal; you can even take turns coming to each other's house in your pj's for wine after the kiddos are in bed.

- **Stop scrolling Facebook and instead call or message your girlfriend.** You know that your 2,000 relationships on Facebook pale in comparison to your #RideOrDie girls. Don't let Fakebook friends take the precious little time you have for the real ones.

- **Be available when they need you.** Remember that it goes both ways. Although it's easy to lose touch with friends when you have little ones, make the extra effort to just show up.

- **Help your children nurture their own village.** Studies show that our relationships as children have almost as much impact on our health as diet and exercise, so help your children create their own supportive relationships.

Hack 108
Make Someone Else's Day

The best way to feel happier is to stop thinking about your own happiness and focus on someone else's. In studies where participants were given different amounts of money, their happiness the next day was not tied to how much they'd spent on themselves but what they'd done for others.[5] You don't have to give money—any action where you fixate on someone else's happiness draws your attention away from your internal monologue.

In the world of happiness, it's fuzzy math: if you focus solely on your happiness, you probably make zero people—including yourself—happy; focus on someone else's happiness, and you get two happy people.

- **Compliment someone.** Starting today, if you think of a positive thought about someone, share it. At that moment.

- **Practice random acts of kindness.** Remember that cheesy bumper sticker from the 1990s? It's not just for hippies: according to a study from the United Kingdom, doing these little acts once a day raised levels of happiness.[6]

- **Hand-deliver a thank-you letter.** Who has impacted you in some way that you've never properly thanked? In a study of positive psychology interventions by Dr. Martin Seligman, participants who personally delivered a letter of thanks experienced increased happiness scores for more than a month.[7] If you can't deliver in person, mail the letter and follow up with a phone call.

- **Volunteer with your children.** Teach your children the wonder of helping others with projects you can do together. Start small, such as a half-day experience on Martin Luther King Jr. Day or another holiday. Not only does volunteering increase their sense of gratitude and empower them to help others, studies have found that children and teenagers who volunteer engage in fewer at-risk behaviors.[8]

- **Allow your children to donate money.** If you typically donate a certain amount every year, set aside a portion for
your children to choose the charity recipient. Your child
will learn a habit of generosity and also receive the happiness boost that comes with it.

Hack 109
Forgive

I'm exceptionally good at carrying a running tally of insults and
slights, like some crazy bad-check ledger. But holding a grudge
doesn't help *you*. On the other hand, research shows that women
who forgive others are less likely to report depression, regardless
of how the other person reacted.[9]

Amit Sood[10] uses the following analogy: When we're exposed
to poison ivy, the chemical urushiol adheres to our skin, triggering an immune reaction. Long after the urushiol is washed
away, our skin is still reacting. In fact, it's our skin's exaggerated
reaction—and not the chemical itself—that creates the damage.
Holding on to anger and grudges is the same—it's not the actual
event that causes the prolonged damage but our response to it.

To quote Nelson Mandela, "Resentment is like drinking poison and then hoping it will kill your enemies."

- **Find commonalities between you and the other person.**
When you're angry, the fast brain kicks in, and you see the
other person as "other." But we're more likely to empathize
with others when we share something in common, so intentionally identifying commonalities allows your slow
brain to kick in. Remind yourself of Maya Angelou's poem
"Human Family": "We are more alike, my friends, than we
are unalike."[11] What do you and the other person have in
common?

- **Remember that we are *all* facing our own struggles, even if they're not obvious.** Once I was in the ER, taking care of a young boy with a small cut, and, no matter what I did for the child, the father was critical. I did my best but silently seethed. Weeks later, we received a letter of thanks from the family, noting that they had previously lost a child, and that, despite their immense fear, we had comforted them. You just *never* know. If you can simply remind yourself that the other person is facing some struggle that you don't know, empathy and compassion come more easily.

- **Plan ahead for tough situations.** You know which situations can trigger your angry self. Maybe it's a get-together with a specific family member or a snide coworker. Before you encounter the situation again, instead of arming yourself with withering George Costanza–style comebacks, arm yourself with these tools for compassion.

Hack 110
When in Doubt, Play

I've seen enough as an ER doctor to know that we shouldn't take one day of good health for granted. And yet, even so, I forget. It can be really hard to just *be* for the eighteenth tea party of the day.

Then my son became so sick with the stomach bug as an infant that I had to take him to the ER. IVs were hooked into his pudgy arm. I sat on his hospital bed, cradling him in my arms as a helpless parent—in an ER where I was so accustomed to being in charge. I yearned to just be able to take him home and say yes to reading *Moo, Baa, La La La* before bed . . . *sixteen times.*

Find activities that you and your family love. Do them together. Often. Celebrate silly things, like Learn Your Name in Morse Code Day (it's January 11, FYI) or Pi Day (you'd better know when that is, friend), as one of my best girlfriends does with glee every year. Because there's no time like the present to celebrate. Even amid the madness of this time, we have much to celebrate, and the more you look for and savor it, the more you will see it.

- **Focus your attention on your child's small milestones.** Notice how he is growing and changing. He's likely doing something new today that he didn't yesterday. Celebrate that!

- **Create a nightly favorite family ritual.** As often as we can, we do family dance party before bath. Right now, my daughter requests Brandon Flowers, *Magdalena,* or anything Whitney Houston. (What can I say? I raised her well.) We're goofy. We have family moves. We laugh. Find something that you love to do together, whether it's board games, singing, looking at family pictures and videos, or whatever gets you laughing.

- **Have weekly family dates.** I have a friend who works long hours and often gets home after her children have gone to bed. But, on Saturday afternoons, she and her children have a weekly tea party. They pull out their finest plastic tea set. Sometimes they drink water or juice. Sometimes they just imagine. What matters is that her children know that she prioritizes her time with them.

- **Don't wait for a holiday to celebrate.** The fact that it's Friday is worth celebrating with family pizza night. Your child got a sticker at school? Worthy of an extra game of hide and seek! One child said something nice about their sibling? *Definitely* worth a celebration of a tickle fight, extra reading time together, or a board game night. The celebration need not be elaborate; fun time together as a family is reward enough.

- **Belly laugh.** Read to your children in funny voices. Have a contest of who can make the best alphabet letters with their body. Belly laugh with your children like you're eight years old again. Laugh so hard that tears cloud your vision. Because it's in these moments that we see our life's miracles most clearly.

Dr. Darria's Restore Diet

*(aka how to lose the weight + recalibrate your body,
when you don't have time to pee in private)*

I get asked all the time for weight loss tips. Now, while I'm not one for "miracle" short-term fixes or just focusing on weight, I know how much I was itching to lose those fifty pounds I gained with each pregnancy, too. But this system doesn't just help shed weight—it restores your body's equilibrium and health, too.

The great thing? There's no counting calories, carbs, fat, or anything else. I'm not just trying to make it "easy"—I *don't* want restricting calories to be your focus. For one, if you're eating the right foods, you won't need to; plus, restricting too much can drop your metabolism, make you miserable and sabotage your efforts.

Okay. Got it? Ready?

The Plan consists of 3 pillars: (1) eating the "Trifecta" at each meal, (2) eliminating sugar and "whites," (3) time restriction. (See the corresponding hack ##'s of each for more details.) *The plan below is for "Restore Mode" to lose weight and restore equilibrium. Once you've reached your health goals, you can switch to "Maintenance Mode, page 245."*

1. Build All Meals from the Trifecta

Fats (10 percent)

Protein (30 percent)

Fruits/Veggies/Legumes (60 percent)

- Whenever you have a meal, make sure that it has ALL THREE of the Trifecta: (1) Produce/legumes, (2) protein, (3) and fats. This combination gives you volume plus satiety, and is crucial to stay full, keep energy levels up, blood glucose level, and cravings down.

- Nutritional guidelines often refer to recommended amounts as a "percent of calories." Since I don't want you to have to count calories, I refer to them as a visual "percent of your plate."

  - **Unlimited veggies, beans/legumes, and fruit (60 percent of your plate):** Eat as many of these as you want in their whole (i.e., not juice) form. Many people feel hungry on diets because they just don't get enough volume. So, take advantage of these "diet freebies" by filling your plate with them. (See hacks #3–6 for produce, and hack #7 and #10 for beans and legumes.)

  - **Protein** (30 percent of your plate): Stick to the "Best" and "Middle" protein sources; think chicken without the skin, fish, lean meats or game meats. (See hack #10 for the total list.)

  - **Good fats** (10 percent of your plate): Just like protein, you want to stick to the "best" and "good" sources, such as olive oil, nuts, avocado, macadamia oil, and fatty fish. (See hack #8.)

2. Cut Sugar and "White" Carbs

Whether it's obvious sugar sources (cookies), hidden ones (salad dressings with as much sugar as chocolate syrup), or "white" processed carbs (white pasta, white bread), sugar in any form is a weight-gain magnet (see The Science of Sugar, page 37). Plus, if you're in a cycle of chronically eating high sugar, your sugar dependence and cravings drive your choices—and will always overpower your good intentions. Time to rewire your brain and body. Pro Tip: Many find it easier to take this tactic: eliminate hidden sugars and "whites" first. After about two weeks, your taste buds will have adjusted, at which point it's less of a struggle to then cut sweets.

- **Cut hidden sugar and "white" carbs:** These carbs immediately convert to sugar in your bloodstream, just as if you ate candy. Replace them with lower-sugar versions (hack #13) and "best" carbs (below).

- **Optional "best" carbs:** You can add "best" carbs (sprouted breads, ancient grains, 100 percent bran cereal) to any Trifecta meal, but limit less than 25 percent of your plate, since these are easy to overdo. Shopping note: ignore marketing ploys, and instead look for phrases such as "sprouted grains," 2 grams of fiber/100 calories on the nutrition label, or the word "whole" early in the ingredient list.

- **Eliminate sweets:** Yes. You will need to cut candy, donuts, and any other sugary treat while you break the habit. Note: Do I mean you can never again have sweets? No! The problem isn't sugar, but that we're *always* bathing our body in it. But first, break the sugar dependence, and you'll break its impact on your weight and health (hack #14).

3. When: Restrict Your Eating Window

This was a cornerstone to losing my baby weight. Even now, when I'm in "maintenance mode," I'll loosely follow this during the week.

- **To lose weight:** Stick to an 11- to 12-hour window (i.e., breakfast at 8:00 A.M., last meal done by 7:00 or 8:00 P.M.). You can try to limit it even more (the best results are around a 9-hour window), although I find that to be difficult with kiddos. Outside of that window, it's water and herbal tea, but no other food. (See Hack #21 for more details and the research behind it.)

- **Cheat!** Research supports that a little scheduled cheating on weekends is okay. Don't go crazy with pizza and ice cream at 3 A.M., but it's totally fine to have a meal or dessert outside of your normal window on a weekend.

What It Looks Like:
An Example Day (*Restore Mode*)

- **6:00 A.M.:** 16 ounces water (and throughout the day)

- **6:45 A.M.:** 1 cup coffee

- **7:30 A.M.:** scrambled eggs with smoked salmon, large serving of cantaloupe, nut-based or dairy yogurt

- **10:00 A.M.:** spoonful of nut butter and a banana

- **1:00 P.M.:** large vegetable salad (don't give me some stingy salad—I want lettuce, tomatoes, corn, black olives, peppers, cabbage—whatever veggies you have), tofu, and black beans. Salsa and macadamia or avocado oil for dressing, and a ¼ to ½ cup guacamole (see hack #6 for my Longevity Salad)

- **4:00 P.M.:** unlimited carrots, peppers, or celery, with hummus or olive tapenade

- **6:30 P.M.:** salmon cooked with olive oil, balsamic vinegar and garlic, half a plate full of roasted green beans and roasted broccoli, quinoa. Plus, another huge salad if I want.

Getting Started

For fastest results, do all three pillars at once. But, if that seems overwhelming, start with one or two. In less than two weeks, you'll notice a difference and naturally have the motivation to do more.

Maintenance Mode

The beauty of this "Diet" is that it restores your health and body's equilibrium, and then is one you can follow for life. Truly it's something you can enjoy. So, once you've reached your goals, make the following small shifts for maintenance mode.

- **Loosen your eating window:** Stick to around 12 to13 hours on weekdays.

- **You can add back more "middle" carbs,** for a recommended 3 to 4 servings a day.

- **Sugary treats:** I know you were waiting for this—yes, of course, now if you want the occasional sweet treat, you can have it. Although you'll likely not want it nearly as much as you once did! Salud!

Notes

A Letter from Me to You

1. www.npr.org/2017/05/12/528098789/u-s-has-the-worst-rate-of
-maternal-deaths-in-the-developed-world.

Part 1: Nutrition

1. www.nobelprize.org/educational/medicine/vitamin_b1/eijkman
.html.

2. McDowell, Lee. *Vitamin History, The Early Years* (First Edition
Design, 2013), www.amazon.com/Vitamin History Early-Years
-McDowell/dp/1622872665.

3. www.jameslindlibrary.org/articles/adolphe-vordermans-1897
-study-on-beriberi-an-example-of-scrupulous-efforts-to-avoid-bias/.

4. Dr. Keith Roach, personal communication, June 12, 2018.

5. www.frontiersin.org/articles/10.3389/fpsyg.2014.00444/full.

6. Charles Duhigg, *Smarter Faster Better* (New York: Random
House, 2016), 30.

Hacks to Set Your Goals

1. Duhigg, *Smarter Faster Better,* 30.

2. Duhigg, *Smarter Faster Better,* 30.

3. Interview with the author, April 1, 2018.

4. www.hsph.harvard.edu/news/press-releases/improving
-diet-quality-over-time-linked-with-reduced-risk-premature-death/.

5. www.ncbi.nlm.nih.gov/pubmed/19880930.

6. www.apa.org/monitor/2017/09/food-mental-health.aspx.

7. www.businessnewsdaily.com/3699-healthy-eating-worker-productivity.html#sthash.nah4BJTh.dpuf.

8. www.consumerreports.org/prescription-drugs/too-many-meds-americas-love-affair-with-prescription-medication/#nation.

9. www.ncbi.nlm.nih.gov/pubmed/12243933.

10. www.ncbi.nlm.nih.gov/pubmed/16880426.

11. www.ncbi.nlm.nih.gov/pubmed?term=23221879.

12. National Weight Control Registry, www.nwcr.ws/research/.

13. www.hsph.harvard.edu/obesity-prevention-source/obesity-causes/genes-and-obesity/.

14. www.ncbi.nlm.nih.gov/pmc/articles/PMC2531152/.

15. https://jamanetwork.com/journals/jama/article-abstract/2673150?redirect=true.

16. https://jamanetwork.com/journals/jama/fullarticle/1199154.

17. www.ncbi.nlm.nih.gov/pubmed/16441938.

The Building Blocks of a Healthy Diet

1. www.theguardian.com/environment/2016/jul/13/us-food-waste-ugly-fruit-vegetables-perfect?CMP=share_btn_tw.

2. https://jamanetwork.com/journals/jama/fullarticle/1199154.

3. www.ncbi.nlm.nih.gov/pmc/articles/PMC4848870/.

4. www.ncbi.nlm.nih.gov/pubmed/27133167.

5. http://jamanetwork.com/journals/jama/article-abstract/2281702.

6. http://science.sciencemag.org/content/341/6150/1241214.

7. www.ncbi.nlm.nih.gov/pubmed/18326589.

8. www.scientificamerican.com/article/how-gut-bacteria-help-make-us-fat-and-thin/.

9. www.scientificamerican.com/article/how-gut-bacteria-help-make-us-fat-and-thin/.

10. www.gastro.org/press_releases/prebiotics-reduce-body-fat-in-overweight-children.

11. www.cornucopia.org/yogurt/.

12. https://medlineplus.gov/magazine/issues/winter16/articles /winter16pg22.html.

13. www.ncbi.nlm.nih.gov/pubmed/22441545.

14. www.ncbi.nlm.nih.gov/pubmed/28192108.

15. http://jamanetwork.com/journals/jamapediatrics/full article/2467334.

16. www.ncbi.nlm.nih.gov/pubmed?term=19307518.

17. https://jamanetwork.com/journals/jamainternalmedicine /fullarticle/2540540.

18. https://jamanetwork.com/journals/jamainternalmedicine /fullarticle/2540540.

19. www.ncbi.nlm.nih.gov/pubmed/24820437.

20. www.tandfonline.com/doi/full/10.3402/fnr.v60.32634.

21. www.ncbi.nlm.nih.gov/pubmed?term=29145952.

22. www.ewg.org/research/ewgs-good-seafood-guide#.WsZ6XRP wYmU.

What Not to Eat

1. www.ncbi.nlm.nih.gov/pmc/articles/PMC4565596/.

2. www.ncbi.nlm.nih.gov/pubmed/26899737.

3. www.ncbi.nlm.nih.gov/pubmed/19339405.

4. www.ncbi.nlm.nih.gov/pubmed/28795605.

5. www.publix.com/pd/white-house-100-apple-juice-all-natural -fresh-pressed/RIO-PCI-104108.

6. www.myfitnesspal.com/food/calories/coca-cola-12oz-canned -regular-coke-211966712.

7. http://pediatrics.aappublications.org/content/127/6/1182.

8. www.ncbi.nlm.nih.gov/pubmed?term=20019905.

9. www.scientificamerican.com/article/bpa-free-plastic-containers -may-be-just-as-hazardous/.

10. www.consumerreports.org/dishwashers/can-you-put -plasticware-in-the-dishwasher/.

11. www.ncbi.nlm.nih.gov/pubmed/17617461.

12. www.ncbi.nlm.nih.gov/pmc/articles/PMC3490437/.

13. http://onlinelibrary.wiley.com/doi/10.1002/oby.21371/full.

14. www.fda.gov/Food/GuidanceRegulation/GuidanceDocuments RegulatoryInformation/LabelingNutrition/ucm385663.htm.

15. www.rwjf.org/en/library/research/2009/10/evaluating-the -nutrition-quality-and-marketing-of-children-s-cer.html.

16. To calculate sugar as a percent of calories for an example food with 10 grams sugar and 160 calories per serving: There are 4 calories in a gram of sugar. So multiply the grams by 4 ($10 \times 4 = 40$ calories). Then divide 40 calories / 160 calories = 25 percent of calories for this food from sugar. According to the WHO, we should aim to keep the percentage of calories from sugar to a maximum of 10 percent, and ideally less than 5 percent.

17. www.heart.org/en/healthy-living/healthy-eating/eat-smart /sugar/added-sugars.

18. www.ncbi.nlm.nih.gov/pmc/articles/PMC4962164/.

19. www.nejm.org/doi/full/10.1056/NEJMoa1014296#t=article.

20. www.ncbi.nlm.nih.gov/pubmed/19815044.

21. www.ncbi.nlm.nih.gov/pubmed/21574706.

22. www.ncbi.nlm.nih.gov/pmc/articles/PMC4742721/.

23. www.nature.com/articles/ijo201369?message=remove& WT.ec_id=IJO-201401.

24. www.sciencedaily.com/releases/2015/12/151211131546.htm.

25. www.ncbi.nlm.nih.gov/pubmed/19071169/.

Make Healthy Eating Delicious

1. www.ncbi.nlm.nih.gov/pmc/articles/PMC4910838/.

2. http://journals.sagepub.com/doi/10.1177/0956797612471953.

Design Your Life to
Make Good Nutrition Easier

1. www.nytimes.com/2013/05/19/health/the-health-toll-of
-immigration.html.

2. www.frontiersin.org/articles/10.3389/fpsyg.2014.00444/full.

3. www.ncbi.nlm.nih.gov/pubmed/21678172.

4. http://journals.ama.org/doi/10.1509/jm.11.0610?code=amma
-site.

5. www.washingtonpost.com/business/technology/google
-crunches-data-on-munching-in-office/2013/09/01/3902b444-0e
83-11e3-85b6-d27422650fd5_story.
html?noredirect=on&utm_term=.431d22b2b46b.

6. www.ncbi.nlm.nih.gov/pmc/articles/PMC4635036/.

7. www.ncbi.nlm.nih.gov/pmc/articles/PMC5388543/.

8. www.ncbi.nlm.nih.gov/pubmed/15465745.

9. www.ncbi.nlm.nih.gov/pubmed/21678913.

10. http://bmjopen.bmj.com/content/4/12/e005813.

11. www.newsweek.com/phthalates-865275.

12. www.nih.gov/news-events/nih-research-matters/friends-family
-may-play-role-obesity.

Getting the Whole Family Eating Well

1. www.ncbi.nlm.nih.gov/pubmed/28818089.

2. www.ncbi.nlm.nih.gov/pubmed/24903612.

3. www.ncbi.nlm.nih.gov/pubmed/25266343.

4. www.ncbi.nlm.nih.gov/pubmed/18180407.

5. www.ncbi.nlm.nih.gov/pubmed/25266343.

6. https://onlinelibrary.wiley.com/doi/abs/10.1002/cd.155.

7. Interview by the author with Dr. Jerica Berge, September 7,
2017.

8. www.ncbi.nlm.nih.gov/pmc/articles/PMC3340527/.

9. www.ncbi.nlm.nih.gov/pubmed/25266343.

10. Interview by the author with Dr. Jerica Berge, September 7, 2017.

11. www.ncbi.nlm.nih.gov/pmc/articles/PMC3663732/.

12. www.ncbi.nlm.nih.gov/pubmed/28632864.

13. http://pediatrics.aappublications.org/content/early/2014/10/08/peds.2014-1936.

14. http://pediatrics.aappublications.org/content/early/2014/10/08/peds.2014-1936.

15. www.rwjf.org/en/library/research/2009/10/evaluating-the-nutrition-quality-and-marketing-of-children-s-cer.html.

16. www.ncbi.nlm.nih.gov/pubmed/24709485.

17 www.ncbi.nlm.nih.gov/pubmed/24709485.

18. www.ncbi.nlm.nih.gov/pubmed/19167954.

19. www.sciencedaily.com/releases/2007/04/070418163652.htm.

20. www.ncbi.nlm.nih.gov/pubmed/28027215.

21. www.ncbi.nlm.nih.gov/pubmed/26063588.

22. www.ncbi.nlm.nih.gov/pubmed/14702019.

23. http://jn.nutrition.org/content/143/7/1194.long.

24. www.ncbi.nlm.nih.gov/pmc/articles/PMC4382151/.

25. http://pediatrics.aappublications.org/content/117/6/2047.

26. https://academic.oup.com/her/article/15/1/39/775700.

27. www.sciencedirect.com/science/article/pii/S221226721600157X.

28. www.ncbi.nlm.nih.gov/pmc/articles/PMC2943861/.

29. www.ncbi.nlm.nih.gov/pmc/articles/PMC2943861/.

Part 2: Exercise

1. www.freep.com/story/sports/2015/06/16/paralyzed-football-player-moves-michigan/28796049/.

2. www.instagram.com/p/BiC2o8YFYLU/?hl=en&taken-by=chrisanorton16.

The Basics

1. www.instagram.com/p/BhucFFmllgG/?hl=en&taken-by=chrisa norton16.

2. http://psycnet.apa.org/record/1998-02141-003.

3. https://academic.oup.com/aje/article/151/3/293/113585.

4. http://n.neurology.org/content/early/2018/03/14/WNL.0000000000005290.

5. *Legally Blonde,* dir. Robert Luketic, 2001.

6. www.sciencedaily.com/releases/2018/04/180404163635.htm.

7. www.ncbi.nlm.nih.gov/pubmed/28319590.

8. www.ncbi.nlm.nih.gov/pubmed/18277063.

9. www.tandfonline.com/doi/abs/10.1080/07315724.2015.1022268#.Vcreq5Oqqkp.

10. www.marksdailyapple.com/19-tips-for-avoiding-injuries-during-sprint-sessions/.

11. www.acefitness.org/education-and-resources/lifestyle/blog/6441/top-10-reasons-children-should-exercise.

12. www.acefitness.org/education-and-resources/lifestyle/blog/6441/top-10-reasons-children-should-exercise.

13. www.ncbi.nlm.nih.gov/pubmed/10707334.

14. www.ncbi.nlm.nih.gov/pmc/articles/PMC4227023/.

15. www.ncbi.nlm.nih.gov/pmc/articles/PMC4227023/.

16. www.ncbi.nlm.nih.gov/pubmed/9929086.

17. www.newswise.com/articles/view/658900/?sc=mwhn.

18. http://journals.sagepub.com/doi/abs/10.1177/0956797617721270.

Finding Time

1. www.ncbi.nlm.nih.gov/pubmed/8963358.

2. www.ncbi.nlm.nih.gov/pmc/articles/PMC4227023/.

3. Interview with Dr. Jerica Berge, September 7, 2017.

4. www.ncbi.nlm.nih.gov/pubmed/9086691.

5. www.ncbi.nlm.nih.gov/pubmed/8963358.

6. www.acefitness.org/education-and-resources/lifestyle/blog/5911
/6-benefits-of-exercising-outdoors.

7. www.ncbi.nlm.nih.gov/pmc/articles/PMC4227023/.

8. www.ncbi.nlm.nih.gov/pmc/articles/PMC4227023/.

Making It Fun

1. www.ncbi.nlm.nih.gov/pubmed/28319590.

2. www.tandfonline.com/doi/abs/10.3810/psm.2004.12.671;
www.sciencedaily.com/releases/2018/01/180110223412.htm;
www.opp.com/en/Knowledge-centre/Blog/2018/January/Does
-knowing-your-MBTI-type-help-you-to-get-fit.

3. http://psychology.oxfordre.com/view/10.1093/acrefore
/9780190236557.001.0001/acrefore-9780190236557-e-210.

4. http://science.sciencemag.org/content/149/3681/269.

5. www.sciencedaily.com/releases/2008/11/081111182904.htm.

6. www.pnas.org/content/early/2013/10/10/1217252110.

7. www.ncbi.nlm.nih.gov/pubmed/26618640.

Finding the Motivation
and Building the Habit

1. www.ncbi.nlm.nih.gov/pmc/articles/PMC3084045/.

2. http://psycnet.apa.org/record/2006-12374-010.

3. www.frontiersin.org/articles/10.3389/fpsyg.2014.00444/full.

4. www.ncbi.nlm.nih.gov/pubmed/21749245.

5. http://tinyhabits.com/.

6. www.ncbi.nlm.nih.gov/pubmed/21749245.

7. www.sciencedirect.com/science/article/pii/S0022103111
00031X.

8. http://journals.sagepub.com/doi/10.1177/0146167299025
002010.

9. https://jamanetwork.com/journals/jama/article-abstract/1866 163.

10. www.tinyhabits.com/.

11. https://cdn2.hubspot.net/hubfs/217817/National/Albert %20Lea%20Case%20Study.pdf?__hssc=233546881.1.15209689 27557&__hstc=233546881.1d5392ba03fc5ed380632c0ec30bdf7c .1520968927557.1520968927557.1520968927557.1&__hsfp =2863915060&hsCtaTracking=cb91cf66-9341-4426-a632-216d5 1bfb51c%7C2a3cd802-9608-4a2c-a338-be14056baf92.

12. http://radiomd.com/sharecare/item/30314-implementing -blue-zones-in-your-own-life.

13. www.sciencedaily.com/releases/2013/01/130124091425.htm.

14. www.ncbi.nlm.nih.gov/pmc/articles/PMC4227023/.

15. www.iwillteachyoutoberich.com/blog/c/15-little-life-hacks/.

When the Going Gets Hard

1. www.psychologytoday.com/blog/habits-not-hacks/201408/want -change-your-habits-change-your-environment.

2. http://99u.com/articles/7248/how-to-use-if-then-planning-to -achieve-any-goal.

3. www.sciencedirect.com/science/article/pii/S019566631000 4630.

4. www.sciencedirect.com/science/article/pii/S0191886910000 474.

Part 3: Sleep

1. www.aan.com/PressRoom/Home/PressRelease/1527.

2. www.huffingtonpost.com/2014/11/18/amy-poehler-sleep _n_6174650.html.

3. www.thecut.com/2016/09/25-famous-women-on-insomnia-and -sleep-deprivation.html.

4. http://sk.sagepub.com/navigator/social-cognition/n8.xml.

Sleep Foundation: Structure

1. www.nydailynews.com/life-style/health/consistent-sleeping
-schedule-tied-body-fat-article-1.1521712.

2. www.ncbi.nlm.nih.gov/pubmed/28649427.

3. www.pnas.org/content/106/11/4453.

4. www.sciencedirect.com/science/article/pii/S235272181730
1432.

5. https://thechimericalcapuchin.com/babybooks/.

Sleep Foundation: Routines

1. www.refinery29.com/2015/11/96707/spotify-wake-up-playlist.

2. www.refinery29.com/2015/11/96707/spotify-wake-up-playlist.

3. www.ncbi.nlm.nih.gov/pmc/articles/PMC4826769/.

Sleep Foundation: Environment and Lifestyle

1. www.healthychildren.org/English/ages-stages/baby/sleep/Pages
/A-Parents-Guide-to-Safe-Sleep.aspx.

2. www.ncbi.nlm.nih.gov/pubmed?term=7632984.

3. https://sleepfoundation.org/sleep-topics/sleep-drive-and-your
-body-clock/page/0/1.

4. www.ncbi.nlm.nih.gov/pubmed?term=22750209.

5. www.ncbi.nlm.nih.gov/pubmed?term=16084719.

6. https://physoc.onlinelibrary.wiley.com/doi/10.14814/phy2
.13617.

7. https://physoc.onlinelibrary.wiley.com/doi/10.14814/phy2
.13617.

8. https://physoc.onlinelibrary.wiley.com/doi/10.14814/phy2
.13617.

9. https://sleep.org/articles/choosing-lightbulbs/.

10. www.nature.com/articles/srep36731.

11. www.ncbi.nlm.nih.gov/pmc/articles/PMC4313820/.

12. www.health.harvard.edu/staying-healthy/blue-light-has-a-dark-side.

13. www.ama-assn.org/ama-adopts-guidance-reduce-harm-high-intensity-street-lights.

14. http://jamanetwork.com/journals/jamapediatrics/article-abstract/2571467.

15. www.ncbi.nlm.nih.gov/pubmed?term=20030543.

16. www.ncbi.nlm.nih.gov/pmc/articles/PMC1978406/.

17. www.uh.edu/news-events/stories/2017/JULY%2017/07242017bluelight.php.

18. https://sleep.org/articles/what-to-wear-to-bed-2/.

19. https://sleep.org/articles/choosing-sheets/.

20. http://news.bbc.co.uk/2/hi/science/nature/435342.stm.

21. www.ncbi.nlm.nih.gov/pubmed/10918859.

22. https://sleepfoundation.org/sleep-topics/can-music-help-you-calm-down-and-sleep-better.

23. https://sleepfoundation.org/bedroom/touch.php.

24. https://sleepfoundation.org/bedroom/touch.php.

25. https://sleepfoundation.org/bedroom/smell.php.

26. www.ncbi.nlm.nih.gov/pmc/articles/PMC4702189/.

27. www.ncbi.nlm.nih.gov/pubmed/23992533/.

28. www.ncbi.nlm.nih.gov/pmc/articles/PMC3370319/.

Relaxation and Cognitive Techniques for Sleep

1. www.ncbi.nlm.nih.gov/pubmedhealth/PMH0072504/.

2. www.ncbi.nlm.nih.gov/pubmed/26055670.

3. https://www.tuck.com/best-online-cbt-programs/#best_online_cbt_i_programs_and_apps

4. https://academic.oup.com/sleep/article/33/4/531/2454654.

5. https://onlinelibrary.wiley.com/doi/abs/10.1046/j.1365-2869.2003.00337.x.

6. https://adaa.org/sites/default/files/Eisenhaur_414.pdf.

7. www.ncbi.nlm.nih.gov/pmc/articles/PMC3060715/.

8. www.ncbi.nlm.nih.gov/pmc/articles/PMC3077056/pdf/nihms260691.pdf.

Troubleshooting

1. www.ncbi.nlm.nih.gov/pubmed/11825133.

2. www.ncbi.nlm.nih.gov/pubmed?term=27136449.

3. https://jamanetwork.com/journals/jama/fullarticle/189099.

4. www.ncbi.nlm.nih.gov/pubmed?term=15700719.

5. www.ncbi.nlm.nih.gov/pubmed?term=25644982.

Child-Specific Sleep Foundation and Troubleshooting

1. www.baby-chick.com/solutions-for-sleep regression/.

2. www.ncbi.nlm.nih.gov/pubmed/1568841.

3. https://news.nationalgeographic.com/2015/08/150828-baby-mammal-size-differences-panda-kangaroo-science/.

4. www.ncbi.nlm.nih.gov/pubmed/8531589.

5. www.ncbi.nlm.nih.gov/pubmed/21868032.

6. www.happiestbaby.com/blogs/blog/the-5-s-s-for-soothing-babies.

7. www.babysleepscience.com/single-post/2014/09/03/Newborns-and-Sleep-%E2%80%93-The-First-Six-Weeks.

8. www.parentingscience.com/baby-sleep-patterns.html.

9. www.baby-chick.com/solutions-for-sleep-regression/.

Part 4: Resilience

1. Interview by the author with Dr. Elissa Epel, June 14, 2017.

What's Your Why?

1. http://www.rjcohen.org/

2.https://www.ncbi.nlm.nih.gov/pubmed/26630073

My Days Are a Blur

3. Stephen R. Covey, A. Roger Merrill, Rebecca R. Merrill, *First Things First* (Miami: Franklin Covey, 1996), e-book, 114–116.

4. www.sciencedirect.com/science/article/pii/S0022440507 000386.

5. Amit Sood, *The Mayo Clinic Guide to Stress-Free Living* (New York: Da Capo Press, 2013), 50.

6. www.traumacenter.org/products/pdf_files/Benefits_of _Mindfulness.pdf.

7. www.tandfonline.com/doi/abs/10.1080/08959285.2017 .1307842.

8. http://selfdeterminationtheory.org/SDT/documents/2003 _BrownRyan.pdf.

9. http://marc.ucla.edu/mindful-meditations.

10. www.jeremyhunter.net/resources.

11. https://neuroscience.stanford.edu/news/why-modern-world -bad your brain.

12. https://news.utexas.edu/2017/06/26/the-mere-presence-of -your-smartphone-reduces-brain-power.

13. www.ncbi.nlm.nih.gov/pmc/articles/PMC5403814/.

14. http://pediatrics.aappublications.org/content/early/2014/03/05 /peds.2013-3703.

15. http://journals.sagepub.com/doi/abs/10.1177/026540751245 3827.

Cracking Mommy Guilt
and Self-Doubt

1. www.ncbi.nlm.nih.gov/pubmed/24643422.

2. www.nytimes.com/2017/05/08/well/family/the-birth-of-a -mother.html.

3. http://journals.sagepub.com/doi/abs/10.1111/1467-9280 .00415.

4. Sood, *Mayo Clinic Guide to Stress-Free Living*, 68.

5. www.thebritishjournal.com/health/researchers-warn-of
-dangerous-trend-as-survey-finds-women-self-criticise-eight-times
-a-day-281-2016/.

6. www.paulineroseclance.com/pdf/ip_high_achieving_women
.pdf.

7. Christine A. Padesky and Dennis Greenberger, *Mind over
Mood: Change How You Feel by Changing the Way You Think,* 1st ed.
(New York: Guilford Press, 1995).

8. www.ncbi.nlm.nih.gov/pubmed?term=24370337.

9. www.ncbi.nlm.nih.gov/pubmed?term=16337009.

10. www.ncbi.nlm.nih.gov/pubmed?term=19074717.

If You're Feeling Overcommitted
and Exhausted

1. http://neuro.hms.harvard.edu/harvard-mahoney-neuroscience
-institute/brain-newsletter/and-brain-series/dancing-and-brain.

2. http://archive.fortune.com/galleries/2008/fortune/0804/gallery
.bestadvice.fortune/7.html.

3. www.ncbi.nlm.nih.gov/pmc/articles/PMC4445577/.

4. Gabrielle Bernstein, *May Cause Miracles* (New York: Harmony
Books, 2013), 167.

5. www.theguardian.com/environment/2016/jul/27/children
-spend-only-half-the-time-playing-outside-as-their-parents-did.

6. www.ncbi.nlm.nih.gov/pubmed/19568835.

7. www.newswise.com/articles/view/690303/?sc=mwhn.

8. www.ncbi.nlm.nih.gov/pubmed/23720230.

9. www.ncbi.nlm.nih.gov/pmc/articles/PMC4167107/.

10. https://bmcmedicine.biomedcentral.com/articles/10.1186
/s12916-017-0791-y.

11. www.ncbi.nlm.nih.gov/pmc/articles/PMC5353310/.

12. www.medicalnewstoday.com/articles/315781.php.

13. www.health.harvard.edu/blog/nutritional-psychiatry-your
-brain-on-food-201511168626.

14. www.ncbi.nlm.nih.gov/pubmed/11148895.

15. www.ncbi.nlm.nih.gov/pubmed/23653077.

16. www.ncbi.nlm.nih.gov/pubmed/28760175.

17. www.ncbi.nlm.nih.gov/pmc/articles/PMC1470658/.

18. https://today.duke.edu/2000/09/exercise922.html; and www.apa.org/monitor/2011/12/exercise.aspx.

19. http://time.com/4966319/exercise-depression-study/.

20. Traci Mann, *Secrets from the Eating Lab* (New York: Harper Collins, 2017), 174.

21. www.ncbi.nlm.nih.gov/pubmed/12783046.

22. www.ncbi.nlm.nih.gov/pubmed/28319590.

23. http://journals.sagepub.com/doi/abs/10.1177/1359105317 691589?journalCode=hpqa.

24. www.technologyreview.com/s/402450/meditation-and-the -brain/.

25. https://news.harvard.edu/gazette/story/2011/01/eight-weeks -to-a-better-brain/.

26. www.scientificamerican.com/article/scientists-find-one-source -of-prayers-power/.

Nurture the Relationships
that Nourish You

1. www.ncbi.nlm.nih.gov/pubmed/17634565.

2. www.gottman.com/blog/the-four-horsemen-recognizing -criticism-contempt-defensiveness-and-stonewalling/.

3. https://greatergood.berkeley.edu/images/application_uploads /Algoe-GratitudeAndRomance.pdf.

4. www.eonline.com/de/news/609218/kelly-ripa-says-having -lots-of-sex-keeps-her-marriage-to-mark-consuelos-spicy.

5. www.nature.com/articles/ncomms15964.pdf.

6. https://greatergood.berkeley.edu/article/item/kindness_makes _you_happy_and_happiness_makes_you_kind/.

7. www.health.harvard.edu/healthbeat/giving-thanks-can-make
-you-happier.

8. http://mcc.gse.harvard.edu/files/gse-mcc/files/parent_tips_.pdf
?m=1448054400.

9. www.sciencedaily.com/releases/2015/09/150901135117.htm.

10. Sood, *Mayo Clinic Guide to Stress-Free Living*, 217.

11. Maya Angelou, "Human Family," *I Shall Not Be Moved* (New
York: Bantam, 1991), 4.

Acknowledgments

There was an exceptional group of people, without whom *Mom Hacks* would never have happened. I thank each of you from the bottom of my heart. You rock.

Nena Madonia-Oshman, my tireless, energetic, amazing agent. You always told me the truth, had my back, and were there when I needed you (an agent who responds when she's in labor is an agent who never gives up). **Dan Ambrosio** and the entire Da Capo family, you recognized that "Hacks" were the best part. Your support was tireless, your feedback insightful. Thank you for taking a chance on this new author.

Dr. Keith Roach, for your brilliant insights, fact-checking, hilarious margin comments, and reminding me that "dads need help, too." **Dr. Tanya Altmann**, you keep my kiddos healthy, you reviewed my book, and you have great taste in shoes. What else is there? **Dawn Whaley**, thank you for your support of working mothers. Your vision, encouragement, and mentorship supported me when this book was nothing but an idea.

Deepa Chungi, you made me laugh (sometimes when I felt like crying), you came up with lines when I was blocked. You tried my hacks, you liked them, and you kept me believing, in even the most exhausted hours. You also kept me from saying anything really stupid in my book. So, Thanks. **Jennie Treadway-Miller**, when this book was barely more than an amoeba of words, you helped give it shape—and soul. **Beth Creswell Wilson**, you didn't know that becoming a housemate meant you'd also be in-house editor and wordsmith, but I couldn't have asked for a better one.

Dean John McArthur, when I was questioning pursuing work in the media and TV, you asked me, "Why not?" You believed in me, before I dared do so myself. **Dr. Mike Roizen**, from answering questions about Zika and my pregnancy (before anyone else knew I was pregnant) to subtitle questions, I am beyond grateful for your unflagging and incomparable mentorship.

Julie, Heather, Kate, Jess, Jackie, Kim, Susan, Melissa, Dana, Shana, and **Mitra**. To **Rachel, Ashley, Anne, Beth, Katherine, Emily, Fannie, Jordan, Meredith**, and **Carmen** (*Pure Posse Forever!*). You're my village. You were both my inspiration and my sounding board. Whatever I did to have you ladies on my side, I must have done something right.

Mom and Dad, no one ever believed in their children more than you did in us. Thank you for that. Thank you for coming to all of my track meets and everything else in between. Oh, and sorry about those teenage years. **Nelson and Allan**, you grew up to be two fantastic men. I'm so proud to call you brothers and friends.

My hubby, **BTG**, you got up in the middle of the night with the babies so I could sleep. You gave me backrubs after days of typing. You see the best in me, regardless of what I sometimes cannot see. Thank you. Finally, **my two munchkins**. You are the very, very best. And you have no idea that every time you refused to listen, refused to eat, or wouldn't go to sleep, you actually gave me ideas for hacks. Thank you for that. I wonder what lessons you will teach me when you are teenagers. But then I guess that's for another book. . . .

Love, D

Index

About the Author

. . . .

Want more hacks? If so, head over to www.drdarria.com /momhacks (password: unstoppable) to join the movement and unlock the bonuses that come with this book. Discover more tricks and tips, connect with me and other moms on their own journeys, and keep up the amazing work that you started with this book!

At www.drdarria.com/momhacks, you'll have access to videos demonstrating many of the hacks from this book, more details on some of my favorite hacks and my playlist, join the Mom Hacks community, and more.

I know you're ready—join me!

Godspeed Mama.

Dr. Darria

. . . .

DR. DARRIA is an ER doctor who likes to keep people *out* of the ER.

Her mission is for you to feel amazing and reach your health goals, without adding to your workload. In fact, she wants to help you not just reach your health goals but to succeed so well that you don't even think of them again. Because good health should never be a burden; it should instead help you *do everything you want to do.*

Trained at Yale and Harvard, Dr. Darria had access to the very best medicine and science but suddenly found herself a patient when she had two health crises. Instead of accepting these diagnoses as the status quo, she committed herself to finding solutions—which she now shares with readers.

Dr. Darria is a nationally recognized media expert and frequently appears on CNN, Fox News, *The Dr. Oz Show,* and *The Doctors,* contributes blogs at sites such as The Dr. Oz Blog, and MindBodyGreen, and is a clinical assistant professor at the University of Tennessee School of Medicine (*Go Vols!*). Dr. Darria trained in emergency medicine at Yale University and received her MBA from Harvard Business School before joining the faculty of Harvard Medical School.

She lives with her husband, two rambunctiously wonderful kiddos, and bullmastiff (their *first* child, naturally) in Atlanta, Georgia.